In Search of the Perfect Health System

In Search of the Perfect Health System

Mark Britnell

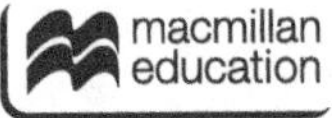

palgrave

First published 2015 by
PALGRAVE

Palgrave in the UK is an imprint of Macmillan Publishers Limited, registered in England, company number 785998, of 4 Crinan Street, London, N1 9XW.

Palgrave Macmillan in the US is a division of St Martin's Press LLC, 175 Fifth Avenue, New York, NY 10010.

Palgrave is the global imprint of the above companies and is represented throughout the world.

Palgrave® and Macmillan® are registered trademarks in the United States, the United Kingdom, Europe and other countries.

ISBN 978-1-137-49661-4 ISBN 978-1-137-49662-1 (eBook)

DOI 10.1007/978-1-137-49662-1

This book is printed on paper suitable for recycling and made from fully managed and sustained forest sources. Logging, pulping and manufacturing processes are expected to conform to the environmental regulations of the country of origin.

A catalogue record for this book is available from the British Library.

A catalog record for this book is available from the Library of Congress.

For Reuben and Beatrix Britnell

'The world is a book and he who does not travel reads only one page'

St Augustine

Contents

Foreword from Lord Nigel Crisp

This book is a masterclass in brief and insightful commentary. If you have ever wondered what was distinctive about healthcare in Asia and the US, what sort of systems the advancing economies of Brazil and Mexico are developing, or how continental European systems differed from the UK and Scandinavia, this book will offer you a short summary of the facts, enlivened with the personal observations of the author. Like all foreign travel this book opens your eyes to new possibilities.

Mark Britnell has filled an important gap here. His unique experience in the public and private sectors, as a payer and a provider, and his great success in leading local, regional, national and global organisations gives his assessments and opinions particular weight and authority. People from different backgrounds will find this book fascinating for the way it illuminates the nature and complexity of healthcare. He shows that healthcare is a social and cultural construct: the health system of a country is a product of history, politics and culture quite as much as it is of science, education and resources. Changing or reforming the health system is therefore as much a social and cultural movement as a business and management challenge. You can't just transport a system from one place to another – but we can all learn from each other.

I have written elsewhere about what we can learn from the poorest countries, and this is represented here by the description of 'jugaad' innovation in India. However, it is the descriptions of countries in the East such as Hong Kong, Japan, South Korea and Singapore that are most intriguing to Western eyes. Their models have led to astonishing improvements: South Korea, for example, implemented universal healthcare in just 12 years and life expectancy has shot up to European levels. These countries are now, however, encountering the health problems of age and affluence. We can all surely learn from their experience and from how they mobilise to take on these new challenges. We can also, sadly, learn from the Russian experience described here in bleak but realistic terms.

Mark Britnell has all the heart and passion of a healthcare professional combined with the head of a man who leads a successful global enterprise. He infuses the book with his own humanity and offers insights forged through experience. Therefore we should all listen when he calls for collective action to tackle the challenges of healthcare and draws attention to the way other industries have collaborated in information technology, communications and much else to develop new and better services. It is a timely and important challenge to us all, and one we must rise to if healthcare is to become sustainable.

Preface

> 'Like all great travellers, I have seen more than I remember and remember more than I have seen'. Benjamin Disraeli. Prime Minister of the United Kingdom, 1868 and 1874–80.

Over the past six years I have had the privilege of working in 60 countries on nearly 200 occasions. I have travelled the circumference of the world 70 times over and worked with hundreds of public and private sector organisations and governments of varying political persuasions. Quite literally, I have engaged with thousands of clinicians, executives and patients from every walk of life. It is an honour to have met so many inspiring people across the world who want to provide outstanding care to the patients and populations they serve.

Three years ago two friends and colleagues – Lord Nigel Crisp, Chair of the All-Party Parliamentary Group on Global Health, and Sir Robert Naylor, Chief Executive of University College London Hospitals – suggested that I capture, in a series of essays, my reflections on the countries I have worked in (but not clients because of confidentiality). This short book, written in a personal capacity, is the result and I am grateful for their encouragement. In between running a global health practice, visiting countries and client engagements, I have scribbled notes and ideas on planes, trains and automobiles at crazy times of the day and night (the only benefit of jet lag) and turned them into a series of observations.

As we all have busy jobs, each chapter can be read in the time it takes to drink a cup of coffee. This is not an academic treatise and has been written for practitioners that have an interest in policy, and policy-makers who want to support better practice. I also hope that patient groups and politicians dip in and out of this book, as well as students in global health.

The 25 country chapters selected for this book cover 80 per cent of the world's economic wealth, 60 per cent of its population and 50 per cent of its land mass. I have chosen these countries because they are both striking and familiar to me. The themes have been selected because of their global importance and the extent they represent common concerns across health systems, countries and continents.

As KPMG's Global Chairman for Health, I prepare for each country I visit through detailed briefings which come in five parts: the political, social and economic context of the country; its healthcare policies and practices; the declared strategy of the system or organisation in question; the characters involved; and the possible solutions required. The job can be pulsating and the time zones punishing but the learning is unique. I have tried to be even-handed with the facts but these inevitably change as the world turns and health services move on. That said, the underlying foundations of most countries' health systems are sturdy and do not shift quickly; it is highly unusual for a country to dramatically change its health status, health service, funding or strategic thrust.

I would like to thank the clients and countries I have visited, the partners and staff in KPMG member firms and the 12-strong International Review Panel that commented on the first draft, which was underpinned by painstaking research from Tanvi Arora and her team in Delhi. I am grateful to Jonty Roland and Richard Vize for drafting and editing advice and could never have entertained the possibility of writing a book without my publishers, Palgrave Macmillan.

As St Augustine says above: 'The world is a book and he who does not travel reads only one page.' If you have got this far, I hope you are encouraged to go further.

Mark Britnell
London, July 2015

1 The Perfect Health System

I have dedicated my entire professional life to leading healthcare organisations at hospital, regional, national and global levels, and am motivated by the pursuit of excellent healthcare. I have worked as a provider and payer and spent 20 years in the NHS. Six years ago I left the NHS Management Board to become Global Chairman for Health at KPMG, a global network of member firms that originated over 100 years ago and now operates in 156 countries.

During my travels I am often asked which country has the best health system and best care. Of course, there is no such thing as a perfect health system and it certainly doesn't reside in any one country, but there are fantastic examples of great health and healthcare around the world which can offer inspiration. In this opening chapter, I identify leading examples that I have seen. I am certainly not claiming I have developed a scientific methodology to inform my observations, but hope I am in a fairly unique position to compare and contrast the good, the bad and the ugly.

There have only been a few attempts to compile global ranking tables on health and healthcare performance between countries. It is notoriously hard to find meaningful indicators and the data is often patchy, difficult to scale or easy to dismiss. The most serious attempt came in 2000 when the World Health Organization (WHO) produced its first – and only – ranking, which placed France on top, followed by Italy, San Marino, Andorra and Malta.[1] It had a substantial methodology but it was hotly contested and highly contentious, so much so that WHO didn't repeat the exercise. Bloomberg produces an annual ranking but uses a limited number of indicators to look at value, efficiency and effectiveness.[2] It places Singapore in pole position, followed by Hong Kong, Italy, Japan and Korea. The methodology is narrow, with only three criteria, but it does highlight the phenomenal success which parts of Asia have achieved in a short time.

The Commonwealth Fund doesn't make its methodology transparent but it does include a much wider and richer number of indicators to judge and rank 11 countries, placing the UK first in 2014, followed by Switzerland, Sweden and Australia, with Germany and the Netherlands tying for fifth place.[3] Finally, the

Economist Intelligence Unit (EIU) also produces a 166-country comparison on outcomes and spending.[4] Once again, this doesn't pretend to cover all meaningful health indicators but it is a worthwhile report which places Japan first, followed by Singapore, Switzerland, Iceland and Australia.

It is a serious and ironic deficiency that in nearly all these rankings there is little attention paid to the recipients of health and healthcare – the patients and citizens. This is a serious omission and it is, unfortunately, the case that no universal patient satisfaction or experience scores exist for meaningful global comparisons. I hope this changes and countries collaborate more effectively in the future.

While countries such as Singapore, Switzerland and Japan feature highly in some of the rankings, it is clear that the range is diverse and the methodologies are different. My search for the perfect health system is much more subjective and identifies examples of great practice which could help stimulate the imagination and effort of practitioners across the world.

The world doesn't have a perfect health system, but if it did, it might look like this:

- **Values and universal healthcare of the UK**
- **Primary care of Israel**
- **Community services of Brazil**
- **Mental health and well-being of Australia**
- **Health promotion of the Nordic countries**
- **Patient and community empowerment in parts of Africa**
- **Research and development of the US**
- **Innovation, flair and speed of India**
- **Information, communications and technology of Singapore**
- **Choice of France**
- **Funding of Switzerland**
- **Aged care of Japan**

Values and Universal Healthcare of the NHS in the UK

The 2012 Olympic Games, held in the UK, were opened in dazzling style and prominently featured the NHS. Hundreds of doctors and nurses enjoyed the privilege of representing the UK's most cherished national institution on a global stage in front of billions of viewers. Polling company Ipsos MORI ranked the NHS first as the institution that made people 'most proud to be British'.[5] Forty-five per cent of people put the NHS top, beating the armed forces, the Olympic squad, the Royal Family and the BBC. Further, 72 per cent of people agreed with the statement that the NHS is 'a symbol of what is great about Britain and we must do everything we can to maintain it'. Its anniversary was ranked first for inspiring national pride (54 per cent) ahead of the coronation of the Queen (43 per cent), the formation of the Beatles (15 per cent), the establishment of the Football Association (8 per cent) and the beginning of the TV series *Doctor Who* (7 per cent).[6]

The NHS was the world's first universal health care system to be established, in 1948, after the Second World War. The first Constitution for the NHS, in 2008, states that 'the NHS belongs to the people' and exists 'to improve our health and well-being, supporting us to keep mentally and physically well, to get better when we are ill and, when we cannot fully recover, to stay as well as we can to the end of our lives. It works at the limits of science – bringing the highest levels of human knowledge and skill to save lives and improve health. It touches our lives at times of basic human need, when care and compassion are what matter most.'[7]

As a member of the NHS Management Board at the time, I was proud to be associated with its publication and believe the British people love the NHS because of its fairness: that it is available to all, irrespective of the ability to pay. A former Chancellor of the Exchequer, Nigel Lawson, once said that the NHS was 'the closest thing the English have to a religion'. Of course, like all religions, change is frequently resisted in the NHS and impeded by shroud-waving.

Primary Care of Israel

By any international standards, Israel has a good health system. In large part, this can be attributed to its excellent primary care, ably supported by four major health maintenance organisations (HMOs). If these HMOs had been based in America the world would have analysed them more. Israel can boast one of the highest life expectancy rates in the world at

82.1 years and one of the lowest shares of GDP spent on health in the Organisation for Economic Co-operation and Development (OECD), at 7.2 per cent. The HMOs act as both purchaser and provider for preventative, primary and community services (some run hospitals too), which are highly accessible. Out-of-hours care is available around the clock and integrated with evening care centres, urgent care centres and home-visit services.

The HMOs all have continuing care and home care units for patients who need help in the transition from hospital back to the community or home and this is reflected by the fact that Israel has one of the lowest proportions of acute care hospital beds in the OECD.[8] Waiting times are low and patients are generally satisfied, with two-thirds being able to see a primary care physician the same day.[9] Great use is made of telehealth and mobile consultations, and the information systems that have been developed in this tech-savvy country are impressive. All the HMOs have comprehensive electronic health records in primary care which support the rapid exchange of information between physicians, laboratories, diagnostic centres and patients. Each Israeli citizen has a unique patient identifier that enables innovative quality monitoring systems such as the Quality in Community Healthcare programme, which encourages a focus on primary prevention. Israel is the only country I have visited where the talk of a 'primary care-led health service' is a reality not rhetoric.

Community Services of Brazil

While Brazil cannot boast a perfect health system, as was demonstrated during the World Cup where popular public anger spilled on to the streets because of concerns over education and health, it has been a victim of its own success to a certain degree through the introduction of SUS (Sistema Único de Saúde, or Unified Health System) and PSF (Programa Saúde da Família, or Family Health Programme). Created by the 1988 Constitution, SUS is one of the largest public health systems in the world and aims to provide universal healthcare largely through the PSF, which is a radical form of community empowerment. While this is seen as a great example for low- to middle-income countries wishing to develop universal healthcare, it can also inform practice across developed nations as the rise of chronic diseases and ageing develops apace. Developed countries need greater 'community activism' to address these pressures.

PSF delivers a nationally scaled model of community services for geographically defined population groups, usually around 4,000 inhabitants. The community teams usually comprise a doctor, nurse, nurse auxiliary and around six community health workers that are recruited locally. They usually serve 100 to 150 households and visit each of them every month, irrespective of need or demand. They provide household-based support for immunisation programmes, chronic disease management, health promotion and screening uptake. They also provide community support for the elderly for conditions such as hypertension and diabetes. Now covering over half of the population, the community health workers have been responsible for sharp reductions in infant mortality and hospitalisations for chronic diseases and mental health problems.[10] While developed countries continue to struggle with fragmented community care and disengaged communities, Brazil offers an innovative solution.

Mental Health and Well-being of Australia

It is notoriously difficult to find global mental health rankings, partly because this critical area of health is still under-resourced in many countries. It is an illness that concerns both developing and developed countries. A recent report by the World Economic Forum and Harvard School of Public Health projected that the global economic costs of mental illness over the next two decades will be more than the costs of cancer, diabetes and respiratory disease put together.[11]

That said, there are countries that are making good progress, including the Netherlands and UK, which both spend more than 10 per cent of their health budgets on mental health. However, Australia has made the most progress in modernising its mental health services from a traditional hospital model where patients are 'warehoused' to a pro-active community system.

Australia leads the way in innovative approaches and has a large number of community services, including crisis and home treatment, early intervention and assertive outreach. A recent OECD report *Making Mental Health Count* noted that the proportion of spending on public psychiatric hospitals dropped from 46 per cent to 12 per cent of the total mental health budget while expenditure on community psychiatry rose from 24 per cent to 39 per cent.[12] Though other countries spend more on mental health in absolute terms, Australia has managed to transform its model of care most successfully to date because successive governments since the early 1990s have made significant policy and funding commitments, including investments in technology. These plans were first started in 1992 with the National Mental Health Strategy and have been repeated every five years or so since.

Australia is ranked first on the 2014 OECD Better Life Index, which measures a number of social determinants that support good mental health: employment, civic participation, education, sense of community, work–life balance and other factors which promote well-being and health.[13]

Health Promotion of the Nordics

While the five countries that comprise the Nordics (Denmark, Finland, Iceland, Norway and Sweden) do not have homogeneous characteristics or national policies, they have similar welfare models where the state plays a dominant role in the formulation of policy for health and well-being. They perform extremely well on the behavioural risk factors associated with poor health: smoking, alcohol consumption, obesity rates and exercise. A recent report from the *Journal of the American Medical Association* indicated that Sweden, Iceland, Norway and Denmark had some of the best rates of smoking reduction, with an annualised rate of decline of 2 per cent to 3 per cent between 1980 and 2012.[14] The Nordics have well-developed public health and illness prevention strategies that are connected not only between national bodies and local municipalities but, increasingly, between the public and private sectors, too. They also seem to have a better blend than most countries between encouraging individual responsibility and fostering collective action from the state in order that both can see what they have to gain from effective preventative care. This has been called 'statist individualism'.

The other distinguishing factor for the success of Nordic health promotion is its longevity. In 2014 the Trondheim Declaration – made between all the Nordic countries – committed itself to 'equitable health and well-being' and strongly supported Health 2020 developed by WHO. This overarching policy framework seeks to address the social determinants of health through four stages: life course, wider society, macro-level context, and governance and delivery. While the themes would be similar in many public health policy statements, the fact that the Nordics first started this type of collaboration back in Helsinki in 1987 demonstrates their commitment to joined-up action between countries, counties, municipalities and a variety of public and private sector organisations and citizens.

Patient and Community Empowerment in Parts of Africa

Given that sub-Saharan Africa only has 3 per cent of the world's healthcare workers but over 25 per cent of the planet's disease burden,[15] it might seem strange that Africa is singled out for patient and carer empowerment. Yet it is precisely because of this fact that countries across the African continent have been forced to innovate by training patients as partners and communities as carers. Once again, given the burden of chronic disease in developed nations, opportunities for so-called 'reverse innovation' abound. Patient empowerment in Africa can deliver better health, improved satisfaction, greater quality and more sustainability.[16] Given the increasingly global shortage of doctors and nurses (estimated by WHO to be over 7 million[17]), all countries could benefit from greater levels of patient activation, which some studies suggest can reduce costs by between 8 per cent and 21 per cent.[18] I do not know of a health system in the world that will not need greater patient activation if it is to become – or remain – sustainable.

I have seen inspiring examples of patient empowerment in Africa, often in the face of tremendous hardship. In Nigeria, I visited the Society for Family Health, an NGO led by Sir Bright Ekweremadu that trains patients and community members in the fight against HIV and TB. Their mission is 'to empower Nigerians, particularly the poor and vulnerable, to lead healthier lives'. Through a brilliant blend of community activism, patient education, social marketing and behaviour change science, their results are impressive. Similarly, The AIDS Support Organisation (TASO) in Uganda trains HIV patients as 'expert clients' who manage drug distribution, home visits, and education for patients and communities. In Kenya, the health minister explained to me the great success of Respectful Maternity Care, which encourages women and mothers to share their experiences with professionals to improve practice and cut maternal and infant deaths.

In nearly every example, African innovation seeks to harness the resources of communities and patients because that is often the difference between life and death.

Research and Development of the US

It might seem odd to juxtapose Africa with the US, the richest country in the world, but it is not always recognised that the research and development might of the US benefits people across the globe. President Obama recently stated that 'now is the time to reach a level of research and development not seen since the height of the space race',[19] and he went on to praise many health and life science projects, including regenerative medicine and human brain mapping. America remains the world's biggest centre for R&D; according to Research America, public and private funding for medical research totalled US$130 billion in 2011–12, more than all of the European Union combined.[20] The National Institute of Health (NIH) is the world's largest funder of biomedical research. In the categories of basic science, diagnostics and therapeutics, the US has contributed more than any other country. While it pays more for this innovation (which fuels the world's highest GDP spend in health), it can boast the largest number of Nobel prizes awarded to its scientists, and the greatest number of 'high-impact' drugs and medical devices developed.

Of course, innovation in basic science, diagnostics and therapeutics has to be coupled with the adoption and adaption of new business and care models. It would be wrong to say that America leads here but it has provided the world with some outstanding examples of business redesign. The integrated health systems of Kaiser Permanente are globally recognised, as is their investment in health information and technology systems. Similarly, Geisinger Health System has offered the world global insights into better population health management and patient care, while Virginia Mason has become a global leader in adapting the Toyota Production System to healthcare. Its lean processes focus on five guiding principles: put the customer first, provide the highest quality, be obsessed with patient safety, achieve the highest rates of staff satisfaction and maintain a successful economic enterprise. The world has learned a lot from these examples but their adoption across America has been limited, although new accountable care organisations are now flourishing.

Innovation, Flair and Speed in India

If innovation is about invention, adoption and adaption then India can claim to have taken adoption and adaption to new levels in a short time. While India has profound challenges associated with the introduction of universal healthcare, its entrepreneurial flair has found ways to provide new services quickly.

In *Necessity: the Mother of Innovation* KPMG highlights Aravind Eye Care, Narayana Health, Vaatsalya, LifeSpring and Apollo Hospitals Group as examples of leading-edge practice.[21] Apollo, the largest provider of telemedicine in India, now claims to have equivalent or better outcomes for medical complications associated with knee, coronary artery and prostate surgery, for example. Many of these organisations treat well-off patients but also serve their disadvantaged communities. This results in a healthy degree of subsidisation while keeping costs down. A case study in the Harvard Business Review concluded that some Indian hospitals had 'developed three powerful organisation advantages: a hub and spoke configuration of assets, an innovative way of who should do what, and a focus on cost effectiveness rather than just cost cutting'.[22]

Many of these hospitals have developed real-time information systems that play a vital role in performance improvement, clinical quality and financial management. They have standardised care pathways which have made task shifting easier so that it is possible to do more with fewer staff. Referral networks channel patients into the right settings and hospitals drive value-based purchasing and supplies to new levels, often manufacturing their own devices or implants, where suppliers have refused to reduce prices.

While people in developed countries do not want Indian levels of health we can learn from their care models and the speed at which trial, reflection and implementation take place.

Information, Communications and Technology of Singapore

When it comes to health information and communications technology (ICT) systems there is no panacea but, as KPMG report in *Accelerating Innovation: The Power of the Crowd*, there are principles and techniques that can increase the chances of success.[23] Great projects create a strategic plan and don't encourage mission creep, put healthcare professionals and patients in the lead, and ruthlessly focus on core elements and build out. In the design phase, organisations use the power of the crowd to accelerate innovation, seek collaborative alignment of diverging stakeholder goals and generate a sense of creative dislocation to make sure ICT systems are not captured by existing practice.

Many of these characteristics can be seen in Singapore. Public hospitals have been sharing patient data since 2004 but the introduction of the National Electronic Health Record in 2011 signalled a shift in gears. Increasingly, all hospitals, community facilities, general practitioners and long-term care homes are linked up, enabling the full analysis of clinical, financial and operational data so that healthcare value can be assessed, because outcomes and costs are better integrated and appreciated. The project has government backing (the city-state is tech savvy) and has taken an incremental approach to the rollout, to ensure that lessons can be learned and incorporated in future phases, stakeholders kept on board and staff trained.

Accenture, in its report *Connected Health*, points to the strong patient focus of the system.[24] It claims that 40 per cent of patients in Singapore can access their own medical information, compared with 17 per cent in America. In its survey across eight countries, which analysed technologies available to patients, Singapore ranked first on every indicator including access to medical records and health-related information, electronic requests for prescriptions, videoconferencing with clinicians, telehealth support and educational support to empower patients.

Choice in France

It is a matter of French pride that their citizens have choice in their healthcare system. *Medecine liberale* is based on three principles: personal payments by patients, choice of doctor and clinical freedom. Patients are free to use any doctor or hospital they wish. They can choose public or private clinics and refer themselves to primary care practitioners, generalists or specialists. Provision of healthcare is very mixed, with about a third of hospitals being for profit, a fifth not-for-profit and the remainder publicly owned. A national programme of social health insurance is financed through employee and employer contributions plus earmarked taxes. The *carte vitale* (a type of medical record credit card) ensures that patients are reimbursed for payments made during care. Reimbursements vary but there are elements of both co-payment and out-of-pocket expenses.

It is important to understand that the concept of choice in France differs markedly from the American-style free competition, the statism of Beveridge or the social insurance of Bismarck. Elements of choice, payment, insurance and clinical freedom have evolved since the formation of the Republic. Patient satisfaction is high but so too are costs. France spends 11.7 per cent of its GDP on health and the system is in some financial distress.[25] Some doctors are demanding greater co-payments (which are not reimbursed through insurance schemes) and there are problems of access in some regions. Policies have been developed to integrate care better and promote the general practitioner as gatekeeper. The reaction to these initiatives has been mixed – as witnessed through the recent strikes by GPs – but it is clear that fragmented care and expenditure cannot continue to escalate, especially as employers face rising costs and the threat of being uncompetitive.

For now, however, patient satisfaction remains relatively high, and quality and outcomes are good. While politicians in the UK defend the NHS and its principles, French politicians have long defended their health system as the ideal synthesis of solidarity and liberalism. Long live the Republic!

Funding of Switzerland

As I have witnessed in my travels, every country faces mounting pressures on its healthcare system. However, the system of Switzerland is the least distressed I have seen. For the Swiss, the old adage 'you get what you pay for' is true. It spends 11.5 per cent of GDP on health,[26] which equates to nearly US$10,000 per person (US$9,276, compared to the US's US$9,146).[27] It is consistently ranked highly and its healthcare system withstood the global financial crisis better than most. Its clinical outcomes are good, patient satisfaction is high and life expectancy is among the best in the world at 82.7 years.[28]

The country can afford such high spending because its economy is globally competitive and dynamic. According to the World Economic Forum Global Competitiveness Index, Switzerland was ranked first because of many interrelated factors including: stable, transparent and effective institutions; excellent infrastructure and connectivity; a world-class education system; a flexible labour market; good stakeholder relations and 'an exceptional capacity for innovation'.[29] The forum cites the education system as being the foundation for its success, along with good collaboration between employers and employees.

While it is axiomatic that almost any health system would be good if 12 per cent of a country's GDP was committed to it, it is important to stress that a sustainable healthcare system is largely dependent on a strong economy. Dynamic countries find a way to harness economic prosperity with a vibrant health and life science sector. Health can generate wealth and, in this light, it is not surprising that Singapore was ranked second in the World Economic Forum study. For developing countries, Singapore is a tremendous system to study because its life expectancy is 82.7,[30] and its spending on health is just 4.3 per cent of GDP.[31]

In both Switzerland and Singapore, sophisticated health insurance schemes have been developed which balance the twin goals of individual responsibility and social solidarity. However, costs, premiums and co-payments have all been increasing and Switzerland has floated the idea of better care integration and a single, comprehensive payer. Remarkably, in a 2014 referendum, Swiss voters rejected proposals for more affordable healthcare because of connotations associated with 'managed care'. Voters have consistently rejected these type of plans. Citizens and patients like what they pay for, although nearly half of the population have signed up for additional insurance with health maintenance organisations. A case of do as I say, not as I do?

Aged Care of Japan

Most people know that Japan's average life expectancy is among the longest in the world, at 83.3 years.[32] People also know that over a quarter of Japanese people are over 65, but few realise its population is set to shrink from 122 million in 2015 to 90 million by 2055.[33] This, when coupled with a sluggish economy and low growth, places enormous pressures on the health and aged care system. I have singled out the aged care system in Japan because it has dealt with its problems head-on and found a good way to care for its elders.

While other countries, such as the Netherlands, have developed good, far-sighted systems, Japan made the bold decision in 2000 to introduce a compulsory long-term care insurance scheme for all. All people aged over 40 pay into the scheme, which offers social care to all those aged over 65 on the basis of need alone. The ability to pay is not part of the assessment process but there is a co-payment for some services of approximately 10 per cent. Japan has a strong tradition of home-based, family care but this is changing as the extended family structure buckles under demographic pressure.

The insurance scheme provides home help as well as access to a variety of community-based services and residential and nursing care. Experimentation has begun with 'nurse robots' in care homes and the technological prowess of Japan means telehealth is thriving. Japan also has the highest number of day centres for the elderly in the world and some of its playgrounds have been modified to provide elders with exercise facilities.[34]

The system relies on national eligibility criteria and uses a computerised assessment process. In this way, benefits can be fairly and universally shared but decisions can be made locally. The national assessment process is supported by a diverse provider market and individual choice. Care managers act as care navigators and provide advice to elders and their carers. As dementia rises – estimates suggest 12 per cent of the elderly population will have dementia by 2020 – 'dementia homes' have been created where groups of people live together in a supportive, home-like environment. In 2004 the Japanese government changed the definition of the word dementia from 'chiho' (meaning idiocy or stupidity) to 'ninchisho' (meaning cognition or disorder). The 2012 'Orange Plan' introduced the concepts of a 'dementia friend' and Japan has managed to mobilise a large number of volunteers in the community.

While this system is under financial stress and subject to periodic review, Japan should be congratulated for respecting its elders and making tough decisions which politicians from other countries lack the courage to take.

Something to Teach, Something to Learn

During my travels to countries with very different cultures, political systems and economies, it has become clear to me that we all have something to teach and something to learn. While it is not desirable to 'lift and shift' health system parts from one country to another, it is possible to stimulate ideas, share possibilities and encourage local innovation, adaption and adoption.

Indeed, many global industries – ranging from defence and telecommunications to energy and life sciences – manage to both compete and collaborate. For something so vitally important as health and healthcare, surely we can work together more effectively for the benefit of patients and populations alike? There are more similarities than differences in most countries' health systems and we should do more together to illustrate what works. As a member of the World Economic Forum Global Agenda Council on the Future of the Health Sector, I intend to play my part and encourage others to do so too.

References

[1] World Health Organization, The world health report 2000: Health systems: Improving performance (WHO, 2001).

[2] Bloomberg, Most efficient healthcare 2014 (Bloomberg.com, 2014).

[3] Commonwealth Fund, Mirror on the wall: How the performance of the US healthcare system performs internationally – 2014 Update (Commonwealth Fund: New York, 2014).

[4] Economist Intelligence Unit, Healthcare outcomes index 2014 (EIU, 2014).

[5] Ipsos MORI, State of the Nation 2013 (Ipsos MORI, 2013).

[6] Ipsos MORI, State of the Nation 2013 (Ipsos MORI, 2013).

[7] Department of Health, The NHS Constitution for England (DH, 2008).

[8] OECD, OECD reviews of healthcare quality 2012: Israel 2012: Raising standards (OECD, 2012).

[9] World Health Organization Europe, Primary health care – Israel (WHO Europe, 2009).

[10] Araujo et al., Contracting for primary care in Brazil: The cases of Bahia and Rio de Janeiro (World Bank, 2014).

11 Bloom D. et al., The global economic burden of non-communicable diseases (World Economic Forum and Harvard School of Public Health, 2011).

12 OECD, Making mental health count (OECD, 2014).

13 OECD, OCED Better Life Index 2014 (OECD, 2014).

14 Ng M. et al., 'Smoking prevalence and cigarette consumption in 187 countries: 1980–2012,' *Journal of American Medical Association*, 311(2), pp. 183–92 (2014).

15 Crisp N. and Chen L., 'Global supply of health professionals,' *New England Journal of Medicine*, 370(10) (2014).

16 All-Party Parliamentary Group on Global Health, Patient empowerment: For better quality more sustainable health services globally (APPG-GH, 2014).

17 World Health Organization, A universal truth: No health without a workforce (WHO, 2013).

18 Hibbard J.H. et al., 'Patients with lower activation associated with higher costs: Delivery systems should know their patients' "scores".' *Health Affairs*, 32, pp. 216–22 (2013).

19 White House, Remarks by the President in his State of the Union Address (White House Office of the Press Secretary, 2013).

20 Research America, Health R&D spending in the US (FY11-12) (Research America, 2013).

21 KPMG International, Necessity: The mother of innovation (KPMG, 2014).

22 Govindarajan V. and Ramamurti R., 'Delivering world-class care affordably,' *Harvard Business Review* (2013).

23 KPMG International, Accelerating innovation: The power of the crowd (KPMG, 2013).

24 Accenture, Connected health (Accenture, 2012).

25 World Bank statistics, Total health expenditure (% of GDP) (World Bank, 2013).

26 World Bank statistics, Total health expenditure (% of GDP) (World Bank, 2013).

27 World Bank statistics, Total health expenditure per capita (World Bank, 2013).

28 World Bank statistics, Life expectancy at birth (World Bank, 2013).

29 World Economic Forum, Global Competitiveness Report 2014–15 (WEF, 2014).

30 World Bank statistics, Life expectancy at birth (World Bank, 2013).

31 World Bank statistics, Total health expenditure (% of GDP) (World Bank, 2013).

32 World Bank statistics, Life expectancy at birth (World Bank, 2013).

33 Kaneko R. et al., 'Population projections for Japan: 2006–55,' *Japanese Journal of Population*, 6(1) (2008).

34 Pilling D., How Japan stood up to old age (*Financial Times*, 17 January 2014).

Asia and Australia

2 Japan
Live long and prosper

There is an apocryphal Japanese story which tells of five old men sitting in their hospital beds talking about their well-being. They had been in hospital for the past 20 days and were wondering what had happened to their friend, the sixth patient on the ward, who wasn't in his bed that morning. 'Where is Keiichi?' one of the men asked, only for another to reply: 'He is feeling very unwell so he decided to go home.'

This Japanese joke has a grain of truth in it. The demographic forces at play in Japan are monumental. Standing at 83.3 years,[1] Japan has among the highest life expectancies on the planet, and the combination of longevity and a declining birth rate means the country is ageing rapidly. Over a quarter of Japanese people are over 65 and this group already accounts for more than half of Japan's health spending.[2]

Japan's total healthcare spending reached US$479bn in 2013, making it the third-largest spender in the world after the US and China.[3] But healthcare only cost 10.3 per cent of GDP in 2013, around the middle of the Organisation for Economic Co-operation and Development (OECD) countries,[4] making it a cost-effective system.

Demography is placing great pressure on the country's creaking finances, as healthcare costs are forecast to outstrip GDP growth for the foreseeable future. This is compounded by a massive decline in population; it is estimated that Japan will shrink by 32 million people (26 per cent) from 127 million in 2015 to 92 million by 2055, by which time 40 per cent of the population will be aged 65 or over.[5] A smaller, older population producing less tax revenue in a sluggish economy is a dangerous combination for healthcare. Japan's ability to confront these challenges will offer important lessons for other developed countries.

Kaihoken

Established in 1961, Japan's universal health insurance system, known as *kaihoken*, has contributed to sustained and dramatic improvements in life expectancy. The rapid increase, which began in the 1950s, has been attributed to a strong and growing economy, assertive public health policies which tackled communicable diseases, high literacy rates and educational levels, traditional diet and exercise, and a stable political environment. Universal healthcare is a treasured principle among Japanese people.

Kaihoken has a number of distinctive features which have slowly percolated through the cultural, social, economic and political seams of Japan. The goal of universal healthcare was part of a wider drive to create a welfare state in the 1950s and 1960s, as the country moved decisively away from the militarised economy of the 1930s and 1940s. Every Japanese citizen can receive medical care from any hospital or clinic – public or private – with a uniform fee schedule for reimbursement applied nationwide through a system of universal medical insurance. The creation of universal insurance reflected the political desire for social solidarity rather than an ideology of competition and choice.

Fragmentation

Fragmentation is a dominant feature of Japan's healthcare system, with myriad insurers and providers and weak clinical collaboration. There are around 3,500 health insurers,[6] divided into municipally run 'Citizens Health Insurance' schemes for the retired, self-employed and unemployed, and employer–employee schemes. All plans provide the same national benefits package, which covers hospital and ambulatory care, mental health care, drugs, home care, physiotherapy and most dental care. Individuals have no choice of health plan and there is little competition as the government sets the prices. It is widely recognised that there are too many health insurance schemes and many are too small to drive the changes which the healthcare system needs.

There is an element of cost sharing, with everyone having to make co-payments of around 10–30 per cent, with some exceptions for young children and poorer people. A safety net caps personal payments by limiting annual household health and long-term care costs.

The government's ability to control prices has been highly effective, reducing costs or marginally increasing them when rates are set every two years. Effectively, the Cabinet decides the total healthcare expenditure and the Ministry of Finance and Ministry of Health, Labour and Welfare deliberate over the details.

There are over 8,500 hospitals and 100,000 clinics (defined as having fewer than 20 beds),[7] which provide around 13 beds per 1,000 people, triple the OECD average.[8] These facilities are overwhelmingly too small, uneconomic and lacking in critical clinical mass. These extraordinary numbers arose because, historically, facilities developed out of physicians' practices. This is reflected in the current ownership structure: around 80 per cent of hospitals are privately owned, and about half of those are in the hands of doctors.[9] All hospitals are not-for-profit. While private corporations and large employers, such as Hitachi, do own hospitals they are not run to provide a return to their shareholders. Almost three-quarters of hospitals operate at a loss.

With so many institutions and beds, staffing per bed is very low while Japan has four times the number of magnetic resonance imaging (MRI) scanners and six times the number of computed tomography (CT) scanners compared with a similar European population.[10]

Doctors work long hours and there are serious shortages in rural areas, a problem the government is trying to tackle. Collaboration between doctors and specialists is often poor, with multi-speciality teams and clinics uncommon. In an effort to change this, financial incentives were introduced in 2008 to improve care coordination, particularly in cancer, stroke, cardiac and palliative care.

The system is undermanaged, with too little attention paid to organising patient access and developing efficient care pathways. There is no clear boundary between primary and secondary care, and no one acts as a gatekeeper between them, leaving patients free to consult any care provider – primary or specialist – at any time, with full insurance coverage.

This unrestricted approach to access is straining the insurance system and encouraging heavy use of healthcare. The average Japanese makes 13 visits to the doctor every year, more than double the OECD average, while the average length of hospital stay is nearly triple the OECD average.[11] Many patients are in the wrong place; people are using hospitals for routine care that could be provided elsewhere, while elderly patients are in acute hospital beds because they cannot get residential care.

The government has now embarked on a radical reform of facilities and pathways. The proposed changes are enormous: a drastic reduction in acute beds and a big increase in sub-acute beds; nursing care beds; long-term care facilities; and domiciliary care services. All these changes are to be implemented by 2025, along with a rationalisation of hospital sites to improve quality and efficiency.

Bold Reforms in Long-term Care

A big step towards providing older people with the right sort of long-term care was taken in the year 2000, when the government initiated a mandatory long-term care insurance scheme (Kaigo Hoken) to help older people lead more independent lives. The scheme is effectively another pillar of social security alongside healthcare and pensions. It marked a recognition that the traditional approach of leaving families – overwhelmingly women – to provide care was inadequate, and that there was an important role for socialised care. Traditionally, public residential care has been stigmatised, commonly associated with Ubasuteyama (a legendary mountain where old women were abandoned) and implications of family neglect.

The scheme is run by the municipal governments, whose task of predicting demand for care funding is considerably simplified by the government setting the prices. The financing system includes money from central government and contributions of about 1–2 per cent of income paid by anyone over 40. The total cost is around 2 per cent of GDP and it is widely admired, providing a comprehensive range of in-home, community and institutional care. However, cost increases of around 5 per cent a year between 2007 and 2011 have led to reforms to improve efficiency and place greater emphasis on prevention.

Mental health services have lagged behind other countries on issues such as patient rights and public understanding, and there has been a powerful stigma attached to mental illness. But this is now abating and increasing numbers of patients are seeking treatment. Japan has the largest number of psychiatric beds per head in the world – to some extent reflecting the degree of stigma – but in the past decade care has been moving into the community as acceptability has grown.

Healthcare quality is overseen by the 47 local government prefectures, which are responsible for drawing up 'visions' covering everything from prenatal care to disaster medicine. One could argue that this means decisions are made closer to community-level, but the small scale means that quality monitoring is underdeveloped, with an over-reliance on simplistic measures such as staff numbers. There is no systematic national collection of treatment or outcome data, and limited oversight of physician training. Prefectures also oversee annual hospital inspections, but rarely do these get to the heart of the patient experience.

Hospital accreditation is voluntary and undertaken largely as an improvement exercise; roughly a quarter of hospitals are accredited by the Japan Council for Quality Health Care. It does not reveal which hospitals fail.

Tackling health inequalities is undermined by a lack of clear leadership on population health. Since 2000, the government has championed a strategy badged as the National Health Promotion Movement in the 21st Century (Health Japan 21), which aims to prolong healthy life and reduce inequalities. It includes targets for healthy behaviours, diseases and suicides.

The Japanese diet seems to be a key factor in high life expectancy, with Japan having the lowest heart disease rate in the OECD and an obesity rate of around 3.3 per cent, roughly a tenth of that in the US.[12] However, obesity rates are creeping up as the traditional diet is influenced by Western habits, and the rates of some cancers are also climbing. Despite its ageing population, Japan has one of the lowest levels of dementia – and of Alzheimer's disease in particular – in the developed world.

The economic importance of healthcare is underscored by its inclusion in Prime Minister Shinzo Abe's plan to generate growth. Deregulation in healthcare is part of the 'Third Arrow' of the economic turnaround plan – structural reform – alongside fiscal stimulus and monetary expansion. The strategy aims to promote exports of medical technology and accelerate approval of drugs and devices. It is seen as a test of Abe's commitment to deregulation. Just like in the UK, the role of the private sector in healthcare has proved controversial among doctors, with the Japan Medical Association warning that nothing must be done which undermines universal health insurance.

Conclusion

Japan has made huge progress over the past 60 years. It recognised the value of universal healthcare to economic growth and social cohesion early on, and its system has contributed to dramatic improvements in life expectancy. It has been radical in developing a new social policy for its ageing population but its demographic pressures and slow economic growth present substantial challenges for the future. Like many other healthcare systems there is a broad consensus on the reforms that are needed but no clear path for making them happen. There is a crowded bureaucracy with numerous hospitals, insurers and prefectures involved but little clear leadership to drive through the reforms.

While the single-price-setting system has many advantages, the lack of innovation between fragmented payers and providers, coupled with the decentralisation of political power, make change difficult. Japan is a remarkable country with great resilience and ingenuity. The innovation and entrepreneurial flair that made it a global powerhouse will need to be applied fully to healthcare.

References

1 World Bank statistics, Life expectancy at birth (World Bank, 2013).

2 Ministry of Internal Affairs and Communications statistics (2014).

3 Economist Intelligence Unit, Healthcare report: Japan (EIU, March 2015), p. 4.

4 World Bank statistics, Total health expenditure (% of GDP) (World Bank, 2013).

5 National Institute of Population and Social Security Research (2015).

6 Ministry of Health, Labour and Welfare figures (2014).

7 Ministry of Health, Labour and Welfare, Survey of Medical Institutions (MHLW, 2013).

8 OECD health statistics, Hospital beds per 1,000 population (OECD, 2014).

9 Healthcare report: Japan (EIU, December 2014), pp. 2–3.

10 Healthcare report: Japan (EIU, December 2014), pp. 2–3.

11 OECD statistics, Doctors' consultations (number per capita) (OECD, 2011).

12 World Health Organization statistics, Body mass index >=30 (% of population) (WHO, 2014)

3 South Korea National pride and global ambition

I recently spoke at the Korean Hospital Association national conference in Seoul. The conference was enormous, with all the key clinicians, executives and officials debating the central questions facing South Korean healthcare. To the Western eye the opening minutes of the conference were quite different to gatherings in Europe. First, the visible sense of deference and respect between the delegates would have left most Europeans bemused and slightly unnerved. Second, the palpable sense of national pride and ambition was evident as delegates stood – hand on heart – for the South Korean national anthem. Korea is an economic powerhouse with ambitions to project itself further on the global stage. These aspirations are certainly reflected in healthcare.

Universal Cover in 12 Years

As part of its plan for rapid economic expansion, South Korea achieved universal health insurance by 1989, in just over 12 years from its initial rollout. Many believe that former President Park Chung-Hee's unswerving focus on industrialisation has heavily influenced both the structure and the delivery of South Korean healthcare, with all its strengths and weaknesses. In 2000, South Korea merged all of the medical societies into one comprehensive single payer, known as the National Health Insurance Service (NHIS). This universal system is financed by employer and employee contributions as well as government subsidies which include a medical aid programme for those in poverty (2.7 per cent of the population,[1] although some consider this an underestimate). The NHIS collects contributions and reimburses providers as well as providing information to patients and administering long-term care services for the elderly.

The system has always relied on high out-of-pocket spending by patients. The government finances approximately 54 per cent of total health spending (the OECD average is 72 per cent) while the remaining 46 per cent is sourced from private funds, mostly out-of-pocket contributions.[2] With fee-for-service payments and no price regulation of un-covered services, the costs to patients soon mount.

South Korea has developed its healthcare system rapidly over the past 30 years. With an average life expectancy of just over 81 years[3] and a healthcare spend of 7.2 per cent of GDP,[4] one of the lowest proportions in the OECD, South Korea has made dramatic improvements in health status through industrialisation, improved water supply, sanitation, housing and healthcare. However, South Korea's population is ageing rapidly; the proportion aged over 65 is set to increase from 13 per cent to around 38 per cent by 2050.[5] South Korea's senior-citizen growth rate is the highest in the OECD, standing at 3.6 per cent per year compared with an average of 0.56 per cent.[6] Like Japan, this growing trend is already putting pressure on funding and hospital beds. Length of stay is increasing and is now the second highest in the OECD (after Japan).[7]

Healthcare spending is growing rapidly, from US$64 billion in 2009 to around US$113 billion in 2015. A new model of care is needed but a number of structural problems need to be addressed if the health system is to be sustainable. This is a pressing issue, especially as cultural values are moving away from traditional Confucian extended-family care to a more fragmented, Western-style social system. Incredibly, the proportion of older adults living with their children fell from over 80 per cent in 1981 to 27 per cent by 2011.[8] It is still too early to tell whether the new Long-term Care Insurance Programme introduced in 2008 will work.

Hospitals in Control

The historical strength of South Korean healthcare is also its potential weakness. It is dominated by hospitals not health systems. While South Korea has transformed its health economy – from one with limited medical infrastructure and fragmented health financing, covering few people, to one with first-class hospitals and universal health insurance – it is the dominance of the tertiary hospital system that is the biggest issue. Can these hospitals be transformed into health systems, establishing effective networks for primary, secondary, tertiary and community care?

At present, around 94 per cent of hospitals and 88 per cent of beds are privately owned,[9] although they are operated on a not-for-profit basis. There are three levels of hospital care: community clinics, small general hospitals and tertiary hospitals. Thirty of the 43 tertiary hospitals are run by private universities while a further 10 (such as Seoul National University Hospital) are run by universities under the Ministry of Education, Science and Technology; the remainder, such as the Samsung Medical Center, are run by corporations.

Liberal patient choice, coupled with a fee-for-service reimbursement system, has produced upward cost pressures. Hospitals rely exclusively on NHIS reimbursement and out-of-pocket payments as they do not receive any government subsidy for their services. So a poorly designed payments system has encouraged large hospital operators to fend for themselves by attracting patients through the continual expansion and improvement of hospital facilities. In the face of an uncertain economic future and a rapidly ageing population this is not sustainable.

South Korea's community-based healthcare is seriously underdeveloped. Public health centres usually provide limited services such as vaccinations and health education while general practice is delivered by family doctors on their own premises. Primary care needs to shift away from being a gateway to complex hospital care towards prevention and working with patients to find the most appropriate treatment for their needs. Investment and policy continue to focus on hospitals, ignoring some major upstream threats to public health, not least one of the highest male smoking rates in the OECD (45 per cent[10]) and the highest suicide rate in the OECD – 29.1 people per 100,000, or 14,160 suicides per year.[11]

Too many South Koreans are arriving at hospital with conditions such as heart failure and chronic obstructive pulmonary disease (COPD) which should have been detected earlier. But low pay for community doctors inhibits the expansion of the community services which are critical to prevention and rapid diagnosis.

Doctors Versus the Corporations

The divide between poorly resourced community doctors and the big corporate hospitals has come to a head with the issue of plans for a major expansion of telemedicine. The Ministry of Health and Welfare sees remote healthcare as a key way of addressing growing demand and the needs of an ageing, and in some cases remote, population. For companies such as Samsung this opens up the possibility of convergence between its IT and healthcare businesses and it is planning substantial investment in health. But the Korean Medical Association sees telemedicine as paving the way for privatising services and undermining the income of their doctors; it claims that tens of thousands of jobs are at risk among doctors working in small clinics. Others see the doctors as putting their own interests before those of the patients.

The Ministry of Health and Welfare has recognised that the care system is fragmented and has proposed improving both primary care and gatekeeping to hospital services. Recent initiatives include the establishment of a formal GP gatekeeping system and a new fee schedule for primary care services, with a blend of capitation and fee-for-service. On top of this, downward pressure is being applied to hospital prices through the annual negotiation with providers. Like Japan (which influenced the structure of the South Korean system), price negotiations are controlled and price increases kept low, leaving patients with relatively high co-payments. This system was designed to allow universal coverage to be introduced without putting an excessive burden on the government as it forged its policy of economic growth.

Perhaps because of the strong industrialisation and tight price negotiations, university hospitals in South Korea are pioneering new strategies for growth. For example, joint public–private Korea International Medical Association has been created to expand medical tourism, taking a bigger slice of a global business estimated at $50 billion. Many South Korean university hospitals have world-class facilities, which increasingly attract health visitors from China, Russia, Mongolia and other parts of Asia tempted by convenient fly times and competitive prices. However, if the larger university hospitals are to feature prominently on the international stage then the South Korean health system needs to pay more attention to improving quality and publishing care outcomes – an aspect of care that is given added urgency by the persistence of a highly paternalistic relationship between doctors and patients.

Conclusion

The creation of universal health coverage in barely 12 years was an astonishing achievement. Single-minded political leadership dragged the country's health system into the twentieth century, ensuring that rapid industrialisation was underpinned by social policies which shared the benefits of wealth. But the price paid is high out-of-pocket expenses and a repeat of the West's mistake of becoming over-reliant on hospitals.

The focus on innovation and technological adoption pushed by the electronics industry will act as a catalyst for improvement which will drive change in both the East and the West in the coming years. But, closer to home, South Korea must rebalance primary and secondary care to ensure healthcare is sustainable and can cope with the mounting pressures from its ageing population.

References

1 Korean Statistical Information Service (2013).

2 World Bank figures: Health expenditure, public (% of total health expenditure) (World Bank, 2013).

3 World Bank statistics, Life expectancy at birth (World Bank, 2013).

4 World Bank statistics, Total health expenditure (% of GDP) (World Bank, 2013).

5 Economic Intelligence Unit, Healthcare report (EIU, November 2014), p. 10.

6 Goldsmith R.L., 'Health Care System Structure and Delivery in the Republic of Korea', in *New Visions for Public Affairs* (Delaware School of Public Policy Administration, 2012), p. 35.

[7] OECD, Average length of stay in hospitals: 2000 and 2011 (OECD Publishing, 2013).

[8] Goldsmith R.L., 'Health Care System Structure and Delivery in the Republic of Korea', in *New Visions for Public Affairs* (Delaware School of Public Policy Administration, 2012), p. 35.

[9] OECD Stat, For-profit privately owned hospitals & beds in for-profit privately owned hospitals (OECD, 2010 & 2012).

[10] Korean Statistical Information Service (2012).

[11] South Korea's Struggle With Suicide, *The New York Times*, 2 April 2014.

4 China
Communist chimera?

> Liao Dan, a 41-year-old Beijing resident accused of conning a hospital out of tens of thousands of yuan in medical fees to save his seriously ill wife, recently thanked those who had helped him. Liao is accused of copying the hospital's seal and using it to make fake receipts for the blood dialysis treatments of his wife, Du Jinling. Since his story made the headlines nationwide, more than 140,000 Chinese micro-bloggers have donated more than 500,000 yuan (US$80,000) to his family.
>
> *From the South China Morning Post, July 2012*

You could be forgiven for thinking that communist China has the world's most privatised health system. Spending just 5.6 per cent of its GDP on health – low by the standards of the BRICS (Brazil, Russia, India, China and South Africa) – China has been playing catch-up.[1] The share of public spending on health as a proportion of total health expenditure increased from 39 per cent in 2005 to 56 per cent in 2012[2] (not that dissimilar to the US after Obamacare has been fully implemented). Private spending accounted for the remaining 44 per cent, more than three-quarters of which came from out-of-pocket payments.[3] Private insurance across China only accounts for a meagre 3 per cent of total healthcare spending and individuals such as Liao Dan, mentioned above, can be placed under disastrous financial pressure during times of ill health. Hospitals will often receive less than 10 per cent of their income directly from government sources.[4]

Surveys show that the incidence of catastrophic medical expenses (defined by the WHO as where a household's out-of-pocket health spending takes at least 40 per cent of their income after basic needs have been paid for) did not decline over the period 2003–11, with an estimated 13 per cent of the population – 173 million people – facing financial ruin through ill health.[5] More generally, it has been estimated that households across China dedicate an average of around 13 per cent of their spending to health. Commentators identify this as the reason for the relatively low domestic consumption of goods and services, fuelling reliance on export-led growth. China needs to rebalance this trend if its growth is to be more sustainable and the fruits of its expanding economy are to be more 'socially shared'. Widespread anger with the health system in the early 2000s, including the SARS outbreak in 2003, has added to the pressure for change.

In response, the Chinese government has taken major steps to improve healthcare for its 1.3 billion people. This is driven not by ideology but by hard-headed pragmatism, with the government seeing wider and more equal provision of healthcare as an important component of social cohesion. As WHO has pointed out, better healthcare provision is also needed to boost productivity in China's economy, for example by enabling the country to cope with the extraordinary levels of migration to cities.

The National Health and Family Planning Commission has overall responsibility for formulating health policy but this is shared with a number of other ministries, notably the Ministry of Finance, the Ministry of Human Resources and Social Security, and the National Development and Reform Commission. The State Council for Healthcare Reform drives the total reform programme, although the governance and administration is highly decentralised, with regional governments having primary jurisdiction over healthcare. In such an enormous country, with a large state bureaucracy, this ambitious health programme deserves great respect.

Epic Achievements

In terms of sheer scale, the changes in China are the largest health reforms I have seen anywhere in the world, and some of the improvements – especially the push for universal access – are demonstrating substantial success.

In 2009, in response to the growing pressures of an ageing population (with a large increase in chronic disease), the rising costs of healthcare and a wide disparity in provision and quality between urban and rural areas, the State Council announced a plan to achieve universal coverage by 2020. This massive expansion of insurance was one of five major health reform priorities, alongside service delivery, public hospital reform, medicines and public health. These were backed up by staggering increases in government spending on health – in the order of $125 billion more over three years.

Improvements in healthcare insurance have been dramatic. The percentage of the country's population covered by basic insurance increased from approximately 45 per cent in 2006 to 95 per cent in 2011,[6] taking about half a billion extra people into healthcare cover – an epic achievement. This includes 99 per cent of the rural population – less than half of China's population now lives in rural areas, signalling the greatest human migration in history. So government action has resulted in near universal coverage in about half a decade. There has not been a reform programme in the history of healthcare that has embraced so many people in cover.

The subsidy for healthcare insurance was increased and targeted to more deprived areas, but although insurance coverage is broad, it is not deep. Some estimates indicate that, after taking deductibles, co-payments and insurance ceilings into account, patients still have to bear more than half of care costs, partly because hospital prices have increased.

The Shadow of Corruption

Progress on the other reforms has not been so straightforward, reflecting some deep and pernicious interests at work. Traditionally, hospitals have largely remained solvent by marking up prices for drugs and diagnostic services. Doctors – who are poorly paid by international standards – have supplemented their income through extra charges, including overprescribing and unnecessary treatment on a substantial scale. This supports a culture of corruption, collusion, poor governance and a lack of transparency in both hospital care and management. Unethical practices such as bribery and unnecessary surgery are a major problem. There have been examples of physicians securing more than half their income through kickbacks.

Anti-corruption measures have been introduced for hospitals, physicians and suppliers, and a blacklist is being drawn up of pharmaceutical and medical device companies engaged in bribery. Greater transparency is an important part of this drive, such as in the pricing of drugs and supplies. The US$490 million fine levied against GlaxoSmithKline in 2014 for bribing officials, doctors and hospitals is an indication that greater transparency is having an effect, but one outcome in the short term will be greater financial pressure on already overstretched health organisations.

Reforming public hospitals is the pivotal issue for controlling healthcare costs, improving efficiency, raising quality and, ultimately, securing better access to decent healthcare. The reform programme has sought to improve the performance and management of public hospitals by introducing pilot schemes which seek to define the role and responsibilities of hospitals, allow market competition and private ownership of state facilities (almost all hospitals are in state hands), align priorities between different ministries and departments, and introduce modern management techniques such as supply chain management, lean processes and good human resource practices.

The Need for Management Skills

On visits to Beijing, Shenzhen and Shanghai, I encountered considerable enthusiasm for these reforms, although this is tempered by anxiety over funding and management support. For example, some hospital directors wonder whether the government will fill the revenue gap if mark-ups on drugs and diagnostic services are abolished or seriously curtailed. Similarly, there is enthusiasm for improving management but a lack of know-how. There have also been problems with tight cost controls, providing a perverse incentive for hospitals to turn away seriously ill patients. For these reasons, it is too early to tell whether hospital reform will prove as successful as universal coverage.

Medicines management was bolstered in 2011 by the creation of the National Essential Medicines List, supported in part by the work of the National Institute for Health and Care Excellence (NICE) in the UK. Evidence-based protocols and formularies have been developed but, again, it is too early to say whether these have worked, partly because of the sheer enormity of the task and partly because no clear performance management or care-quality regulatory framework exists.

Primary care remains underdeveloped, which leads to large hospitals such as the major academic health centres being overcrowded, especially in large cities. The government aims to relieve the pressure on large hospitals by improving community health centres and county-level hospitals. Primary care providers (community health centres and township health centres) are receiving support to deliver a defined package of basic public health services, and have an emerging role as gatekeepers to prevent the uncontrolled use of expensive hospital services. But making this work will be difficult because people know they are likely to get better treatment in the bigger hospitals. That is where most of the investment and technology is concentrated, which in turn attracts the best doctors and the highest-paying patients.

Like many countries, China faces a pressing shortage of health workers. The huge increase in rural insurance cover has pushed up demand, but the low pay for rural doctors, limited career options and lack of research facilities mean there are too few doctors in the countryside. This has opened up huge disparities in services compared with the affluent east coast. Overall, the reform programme has led to a jump in hospital bed use from 36 per cent to 88 per cent between 2003 and 2011.[7] The government has set an ambition to train approximately 300,000 primary care doctors between 2010 and 2020.[8] Training such huge numbers to the right standard will be immensely difficult. China will need to modernise its approach to care pathway design, workforce development and the allocation of tasks between different types of clinician – especially nurses, who are undervalued.

China has a long way to go in using clinical pathways to increase efficiency and quality. Most secondary and tertiary hospitals have only started using them in the last few years. The next stage will be to expand their use for patients with comorbidities, and combining them with hospital information systems and performance evaluation. At present there is virtually no independent tracking of health outcomes.

In August 2014, China announced that entirely foreign-funded hospitals were planned in seven cities and provinces. This potentially is an important policy change because, previously, foreign investors interested in the hospital sector had to establish joint ventures with Chinese companies. However, the involvement of a number of government agencies in healthcare regulation and overseas investment means there is considerable uncertainty over exactly how this new approach might work.

Hundreds of Millions of Elderly

According to the United Nations, one-third of China's population will be aged over 60 years by 2050, more than double the current number of 178 million.[9] One of the major reasons for this rapidly ageing population is the country's one-child policy. This results in one child having to support two parents as well as grandparents. Some relaxation to the one-child policy is being introduced, but it is unlikely to have a significant impact on fertility rates.

Apart from the human issues, the huge and growing proportion of elderly people presents a formidable economic challenge. To address this, the government has increasingly been focusing on preventing chronic diseases and expanding long-term care. Initiatives include increasing community health provision, establishing additional primary care centres and improving the training of healthcare staff, particularly in poorer parts of the country such as Tibet and Xinjiang province. Other steps taken by the government to promote long-term care include fining children who fail to look after their parents – a move which sits uncomfortably with greater labour mobility – and allowing insurance companies to invest in senior housing.

Average life expectancy rose from 68 years in 1990 to 75.4 years in 2013,[10] with infant mortality more than halving twice over the same period (from 50 per 1,000 live births to 11 per 1,000).[11] The leading cause of death in China is cancer, which in 2011 accounted for around 28 per cent of deaths. Lung cancer is the most prevalent of fatal cancers,[12] unsurprising for a country with an estimated 300 million smokers who between them consume about a third of the world's tobacco.[13] Heart disease, cerebrovascular disease and respiratory diseases are other major causes of mortality – in total WHO estimates that one million Chinese people die every year as a result of tobacco-related disease.[14] The appalling levels of pollution in many cities are exacerbating many serious diseases. Demand for care and medical support continues to grow with the proliferation of chronic conditions such as diabetes and hypertension as lifestyles change and the population ages.

Traditional Chinese medicine continues to play a significant role in the Chinese healthcare system, accounting for as much as 40 per cent of healthcare delivered, according to some sources.[15] Despite their fundamentally different theoretical foundations, traditional and Western medicine are often closely integrated within healthcare providers from clinics to tertiary hospitals, creating a uniquely Chinese understanding of health and healthcare. Dual-qualified practitioners are common. The government takes a supportive approach to traditional medicine, investing in research and promotion, but there are doubts about whether its role will increase or decrease as Western primary care becomes more affordable and available.[16]

Conclusion

China has the money and motivation to expand healthcare coverage and quality but it will need to give greater thought to developing its healthcare leadership capacity and capability if it is not to waste time, effort and resources. China's amazing economic growth has been based on global trade and an open-minded approach to global ideas. These forces will now need to be applied to its domestic healthcare system if progress is to be sustained.

References

1 World Bank statistics, Total health expenditure (% of GDP) (World Bank, 2013).

2 World Bank statistics: Health expenditure, public (% of total health expenditure) (World Bank, 2005 & 2012).

3 World Bank statistics: Out-of-pocket health expenditure (% of private health expenditure on health) (World Bank, 2012).

4 China Center for Health Economics Research, Global hospital management survey – China: Management in healthcare report (Peking University: Beijing, 2014).

5 Meng Q.L. et al., Trends in access to health services and financial protection in China between 2003 and 2011: A cross-sectional study in *The Lancet*, 379 (9818): 805–14 (2012).

6 Economic Intelligence Unit, Healthcare report (EIU, August 2014), p. 4.

7 Huang Y., What money failed to buy: The limits of China's healthcare reform in *Forbes Asia* (Forbes, 3 April 2014).

8 *China Daily*, China plans to train 300,000 general practitioners (*China Daily Press*, 2 April 2010).

9 Liu T. and Sun L., 'An apocalyptic vision of ageing in China: Old age care for the largest elderly population in the world,' in *Zeitschrift für Gerontologie und Geriatrie*, 48 (4) 354–64 (2015).

10 Economic Intelligence Unit, Healthcare report (EIU, August 2014).

11 World Bank statistics, Infant mortality rate (per 1,000 live births) (World Bank, 2013).

12 EIU (2014).

13 World Health Organization Western Pacific Region, Tobacco in China Factsheet (WHO, 2010).

14 WHO (2010).

15 Jia Q., Traditional Chinese Medicine could make 'Health for One' true (World Health Organization, 2005).

16 Xu J. and Yang Y., 'Traditional Chinese Medicine in the Chinese healthcare system,' *Health Policy* 90 (2–3), 133–9 (2009).

5 Hong Kong Demography, democracy and destiny

On the surface, Hong Kong's healthcare system is arguably one of the most efficient in the world. The Special Administrative Region of China boasts one of the highest life expectancies in the world[1] (80 years for men and 86 years for women) while around 6 per cent of GDP is committed to health.[2]

However, deeper analysis reveals that the health system for a population of 7.1 million faces big challenges in the coming years, and major reforms are on their way. A heady combination of demographic and democratic pressures may well reshape the destiny of the Hong Kong health system over the next decade.

Efficient But Expensive

Hong Kong has a dual-track healthcare system; around 90 per cent of acute and 30 per cent of primary care is delivered by the public system, and the rest is private.[3] Despite the overwhelming majority being delivered by the public system, expenditure is split evenly between the two. This makes the public system probably the most efficient in the world, while the private sector is relatively costly.

Under the public health system, public clinics and hospitals offer largely free treatment (with very small co-payments) to anyone with a Hong Kong identity card and to resident children under the age of eleven. There are fees for some services and drugs. Most primary services are overseen by the Department of Health, while the Hong Kong Hospital Authority is a statutory, independent body responsible for all public hospital services and some primary and community care. It manages around 41 public hospitals and 122 specialist and general clinics and employs over 60,000 staff.[4]

Established in 1991, the Hospital Authority has delivered better care and better hospitals, which is particularly impressive given the legacy it inherited. In the early 1990s, the bulk of health spending was accounted for by the private sector, but enormous government support since then has seen the public sector now account for well over half of all spending; between 2007 and 2011 public spending on health increased by 30 per cent in real terms.

Hong Kong's public spending is low, so health accounts for a big proportion; the government estimated that healthcare would account for around 17 per cent of government expenditure in 2014–15, the biggest single area of spending. The government has identified medical services as one of the six growth areas where Hong Kong feels it enjoys an advantage over neighbouring countries. Government initiatives to help the sector include building new public hospitals, upgrading existing ones, improving clinical training and promoting traditional Chinese medicine.

The Hospital Authority only developed its first strategic plan in 2009,[5] which signalled increased spending on clinical services, staff and facilities and paved the way for significant capital investment. Its stated mission is 'Healthy People, Happy Staff, and Trusted by the Community'. It continually faces the glare of the media and is seen as a 'bell-weather' for the development of Hong Kong, so what it does and how it is perceived matters to people and politicians locally and in mainland China.

Pressures are being felt across the health system. While the population is expected to increase by about 5 per cent to 7.6 million between 2014 and 2020,[6] it is the increasing elderly population that is driving hospital demand. The proportion of people aged over 65 is forecast to grow from 14 per cent in 2013 to 18 per cent by 2018,[7] and the prevalence of long-term conditions is expected to jump by almost a third during this period. While the absolute percentage of people over 65 is modest by Western standards, the Hospital Authority reports that the elderly account for over half of all hospital bed days and notes that the average cost of treatment for an elderly patient is 57 per cent higher than for a non-elderly patient.

The leading causes of death today mirror those in the West: cancer, heart disease and respiratory illness. In addition, Hong Kong's position as a global travel and trade hub increases the risk of communicable diseases arriving from other countries, notably China, and this can impose severe strains on the healthcare system. Recent outbreaks include severe acute respiratory syndrome (SARS) and avian influenza (bird flu), as well as swine flu. The Hospital Authority has responded well to these challenges in the past and remains ever-alert to future pandemics.

A further pressure faced by the Hospital Authority has been in maternity services, as mothers from mainland China cross the border to give birth in order to secure Hong Kong nationality for their child. In 2011 nearly half of all newborn babies in Hong Kong were born to mainland-Chinese mothers,[8] causing significant local concern. The government has now effectively banned this form of internal health tourism, in the process depriving private hospitals of a lucrative source of income while saving the public system a cost for which it was not being reimbursed.

Waiting times are a significant problem. Routine outpatient and elective care waiting times in the public sector are increasing. The average waiting time for cataract surgery is around 22 months,[9] and many months of waiting is not uncommon for gynaecology services. Overall, thousands of patients experience waiting times that amount to years.

Keeping Out Foreign Staff

All this increased demand is putting pressure on facilities and staff. A widely recognised shortage of doctors and nurses is being compounded by retirements. Hong Kong has around 1.7 doctors per 1,000 people, less than half that of Germany and even lower than that of thinly staffed Japan.[10] The problem has been exacerbated by almost insurmountable barriers to entry for overseas doctors: only 11 foreign-qualified doctors currently work in the public hospital system.[11] To protect the power of the country's own doctors, the Medical Council requires overseas doctors who want a permanent registration to pass a three-part exam and serve a 12-month internship. This blatant attempt to keep out foreign staff must surely change. As a global financial hub, Hong Kong is happy to see a worldwide flow of finance and this should be reciprocated with the greater movement of medical staff in the future.

New models of care are also expected to increase demand for allied health professionals. Hong Kong's plans to increase the number of doctors, nurses and therapists in training will take time, while the battle for well-qualified and trained staff throughout Asia will intensify over the next decade.

Traditional medicine retains a significant place in the healthcare system, with over 6,000 registered Chinese medicine practitioners[12] – almost half the number of doctors.[13] Treatments include acupuncture and herbal medicines. Around a fifth of medical consultations are provided by traditional Chinese medicine practitioners and they constitute the principal alternative to Western-style primary care.

Like other parts of the world, patients are expecting more. While around 80 per cent of public patients rate their care 'excellent, very good or good'[14] there are concerns about the quality of care, communication, discharge processes and care at home. Once-grateful patients now dare to complain, a phenomenon to which the system is only just beginning to adapt.

The Hospital Authority's Strategy

The Hospital Authority's strategy for 2012 to 2017, called Consolidating for Health, was drawn up after extensive consultations and focuses on four areas: improving the availability of clinical staff; improving quality and safety; maximising efficiency; and enhancing corporate governance and risk management.[15]

The strategy is a solid piece of work that grasps the key trends but it is light on implementation and needs more emphasis on new models of care. The initial concentration on building up public hospitals was the right course of action 20 years ago but many of the diseases that Hong Kong faces today can be treated in different settings, as other countries are demonstrating. In one sense, asking a

Hospital Authority to changes its focus is difficult but it will need to concentrate on developing community care, primary care and home care, all facilitated and accelerated by e-health.

The Hospital Authority has already developed some excellent information systems such as HARPIE, which provides nurse-led assisted care for patients after they have been discharged. This technology could alleviate some workforce pressures by reshaping traditional staff roles. The government's development of an e-health record-sharing platform will encourage collaboration between private and public providers and acute and primary care services.

The weakness of primary care threatens to swamp hospital services over the next decade; the strategy is in danger of being overtaken by the sheer force of demography and the increasing democratisation of expectation. The government currently provides around 90 per cent of total bed days[16]; many believe that leaving private hospitals to provide just 10 per cent of inpatient days is unsustainable.

The Push for Private Insurance

In response to the pressures on healthcare, the government has been preparing the launch of the Voluntary Health Insurance Scheme, which would encourage individuals to use private insurance to supplement state healthcare provision. The government's role would be to regulate plans offered under the scheme while promoting transparency, standardisation and access. So, as with Chinese healthcare, reforms look set to encourage greater use of private health insurance and provision.

The idea is loosely based on the local retirement saving plan, the Mandatory Provident Fund. While there are legitimate concerns that the scheme could represent a move away from free healthcare, the introduction of new insurance offerings might go some way to redress the balance between public and private provision. The average premium is likely to be around HK$4,000 (US$515) per year, which would make premiums some of the highest in the world. So the challenge will be motivating people who are currently receiving 'free' care to take up costly health insurance. The government has set aside HK$50 billion (US$6.4 billion) to smooth the transition to the new scheme by subsidising the cost. Having both one of the most efficient and one of the most costly systems in the world makes it difficult to rebalance health provision between the public and private sectors. It is hard to see how this reform is going to work without more consultation, investment and deliberation.

A pilot scheme providing vouchers to encourage patients over 70 to use private primary care facilities is now being extended across Hong Kong. The annual value of the vouchers is around US$260 per person, double the value used in the pilot.

Conclusion

Voluntary insurance and vouchers could increase the role of the private sector in Hong Kong's healthcare system, but it is too early to tell, and the impact will probably not be enough. Further, this will not be sufficient to overcome the challenges of chronic staff shortages, growing waiting lists and mounting public expectations. There is an urgent need to develop new models of care and shift services away from hospitals if this great health system and wonderfully vibrant city state are to stay ahead.

References

1 World Bank statistics, Life expectancy at birth (World Bank, 2013).

2 Economic Intelligence Unit, Healthcare Report Hong Kong (EIU, May 2014), p. 2.

3 Food and Health Bureau, Your Health, Your life: Consultation document on healthcare reform (Hong Kong SAR Government, 2008), p. 121.

4 Leung P.Y. et al., Sustaining quality, performance and cost-effectiveness in a public hospital system. Presentation available at http://www.ha.org.hk/upload/presentation/347.pdf.

5 Hong Kong Hospital Authority, Helping People Stay Healthy: Strategic Service Plan 2009–2012 (HKHA, 2009).

6 Department of Census and Statistics, Hong Kong population projections: 2012–2041 (Hong Kong SAR Government, 2012), p. 7.

7 Economic Intelligence Unit, Healthcare Report: Hong Kong (EIU, May 2014), p. 10.

8 Economic Intelligence Unit, Healthcare Report: Hong Kong (EIU, May 2014), p. 10.

9 *South China Morning Post*, Strain on Hong Kong's health system increases as government dithers over reform, (South China Morning Post, 22 June 2014).

10 Economist Intelligence Unit, Healthcare Report: Hong Kong (EIU, May 2014), p. 10.

11 Tsang E., Foreign doctors quit Hong Kong public hospitals over licence red tape (*South China Morning Post*, 20 October 2014).

12 *China Daily*, Hong Kong preparing to introduce TCM to the World (*China Daily*, 15 October 2009).

13 Department of Health, Health facts of Hong Kong – 2014 edition (Hong Kong SAR Government, 2014).

14 Hong Kong Hospital Authority, Hospital-based patient experience and satisfaction survey 2013 (Hong Kong SAR Government, 2013).

15 Hong Kong Hospital Authority, Consolidating for health: Strategic plan 2012–2017 (HKHA, 2012).

16 Food and Health Bureau, Your Health, Your Life: Consultation document on healthcare reform (Hong Kong SAR Government, 2008), p. 121.

6 Malaysia
Reform some time, soon?

Anybody who has scaled the magnificent heights of the 88-floor Petronas Towers in Kuala Lumpur will get a good sense of Malaysia's ambition and its desire to become a major economic force in Asia and globally. The story of the building's construction is testimony to the ambition of the government, which has been led by the United Malays National Organisation (UMNO) since it gained independence from Britain in 1957. It wanted construction completed within six years, so it stimulated competition by awarding contracts to two companies – the west tower to a Japanese company and the east tower to a South Korean consortium led by Samsung, which eventually won the race to get to the top. Malaysia needs to adopt a similarly bold approach in healthcare.

Health reform has been mooted for the past 30 years and seriously considered again in the government publication of *1Care for 1Malaysia* in 2009,[1] which promoted the concept of 1Care as a comprehensive, universal national health system for Malaysia's 30 million citizens, supported through the 'spirit of solidarity and equity'. This would replace Malaysia's current two-tier system which provides only basic care for the general population while a thriving private sector caters for individuals and corporations that can afford it. It is argued that the development of a new national health system would strengthen national unity and support Malaysia's ambition to move from being a lower–middle income country to an upper–middle income one through the development of improved infrastructure and a skilled workforce.

There has been rapid progress in the health status of Malaysia since independence. Life expectancy at birth has increased from 59 years in 1957 to 75 years in 2013[2] while infant mortality has fallen from roughly 75 per 1,000 live births to 7 per 1,000 during the same period.[3] Malaysia spends 4 per cent of its GDP on healthcare.[4] In 2005 public health spending overtook private spending for the first time,[5] although private spending is likely to start catching up as a result of growing disposable income of a rising middle class. More than three-quarters of this private spending is 'out of pocket' because the take-up of medical insurance remains low,[6] although there are signs that company and insurance schemes are growing.

The government subsidises public healthcare, which is largely free at the point of delivery or provided at low cost, but provision is skewed towards urban areas, and public facilities are under constant pressure from high demand. In 2011 there was one doctor for every 400 people in Kuala Lumpur, but only one per 3,000 people in rural areas of Borneo.[7] Public hospitals often seem overcrowded and treatment waits can be long, encouraging those who can afford it to turn to the private sector. Administrative control of government health services is highly centralised, with the Ministry of Health maintaining a tight grip on the public system – a remnant of the 1950s British NHS that Malaysia's system was originally based on.

The Longest Health Policy Gestation in History?

The government knows this patchwork system is unsustainable but it has failed to build a clear rationale and consensus for change. Its reform programme has had one of the longest gestation periods I have ever seen, with the 2009 *1Care for 1Malaysia* document still government policy but without sufficient detail or drive to realise it. The document itself spells out this inertia, stating that 'efforts to study the sustainability and eventual introduction of a suitable financing scheme to replace the present one began in the 1980s, to date they have not led to substantive action. Various reasons may have contributed to the inertia such as timing, political will, and readiness of the government, people's acceptance and enabling infrastructure to accommodate the change.'[8]

The reforms proposed by 1Care include the launching of a single social health insurance-based system which would bring together access to government and private providers. Funding for the health insurance would be split equally between general taxation and employer–employee levies and make up around 62 per cent of total health spending, with the remainder coming from private spending (23 per cent) and government-funded public health schemes (15 per cent). These funds would be managed by a non-profit third-party payer: the National Health Financing Authority. The Ministry of Health would give up direct control of government providers and move to a market management and regulation function. A capitated system of primary care would be introduced and value-based payments implemented for other providers to incentivise quality improvement.

In discussion with the (now former) Minister of Health and his officials, it was clear to me that the government intended to consult as widely as possible on its proposals. This 'big tent' approach is partly a political tactic to deny the opposition political ammunition and partly a way to encourage private sector providers, doctors and other stakeholders to see universal coverage as an opportunity rather than a threat. Years later, however, the medical profession remains split, opposition on the financing side has not shifted and the once conservative-sounding deadline of 2020 for the new system to be in operation seems an increasingly ambitious aspiration.

Behind many of the concerns with 1Care lie deeper reservations about the transparency of government and its ability to manage change and to develop systems that use public money effectively. Running through the *1Care for 1Malaysia* document is the issue of legitimacy and trust. Episodes of corruption have undermined belief that any new national social health insurance fund would be administered fairly, transparently and efficiently. Further, the determination of Malaysia to push ahead with economic growth and reform makes some politicians nervous that a rise in contributions from citizens (to part-fund national health insurance) would slow consumption while a rise in contributions from employers would slow investment. The lack of independent economic modelling behind the proposals mean the case for a thriving health system driving growth has not been sufficiently well established.

The Private Healthcare System

Malaysia is proud of its mixed healthcare market and competitive private sector and has identified medical tourism as a key area for growth. International patient numbers doubled between 2007 and 2013 and currently stand at around one million foreigners visiting the more than 200 private hospitals each year.[9] To encourage medical tourism the government has set up the Health Travel Council to promote private hospitals abroad. Tax breaks have been introduced for hospitals running medical tourism programmes and other incentives have been provided to help hospitals expand their facilities. Many are located in high-end beach resorts.

But tax is also having a less benign impact on the cost of private Malaysian healthcare. The rollout in 2015 of the Goods and Services Tax looks likely to be levied on private doctors, despite assurances to the contrary. With anything up to 70 per cent of patients' medical bills in private hospitals made up of doctors' fees, the impact could be substantial.

Recently, Singapore health insurance companies have permitted the treatment of their policyholders in Malaysia, dramatically reducing the price for Singapore while boosting Malaysia's inward investment. Singapore, Indonesia, Japan and China form the bedrock of Malaysia's international patients, but Malaysia also serves the Middle East and, increasingly, North America and Europe.

As the domestic private sector has grown, healthcare provision has also become more international. While healthcare will always reflect national boundaries, cultures and political systems, there is now a trend for some Asian operators to establish hospital chains over multiple territories. HCA in America is known as the largest private hospital group in the world, but the recent highly successful stock market launch of the Malaysian company IHH Healthcare signals a new phase of development coming from the East. IHH operates hospitals, medical centres and clinics in Malaysia, Singapore, China, India, Hong Kong,

Vietnam, Macedonia, Brunei and Turkey and has ambitious plans to accommodate middle-class aspirations for better healthcare across Asia. Speaking to the senior management of the IHH group, it was evident that they wish to set new standards in operating models, quality, information technology and consumer service.

Like many countries in the region, Malaysia's public healthcare services are short of staff. The robust growth in the private sector has helped create a steady flow of experienced staff out of public hospitals and is tending to give the private sector a disproportionate share of specialists. Malaysian medical staff are also emigrating to countries such as Singapore.

Conflicts of Interest

A complicating factor in Malaysia's healthcare system is that government agencies have recently acquired large stakes in healthcare companies. The Johor state government, for example, has a significant stake in a large chain of private hospitals while the federal government's sovereign wealth fund (Khazanah) has a stake in another major provider. Government-linked companies now account for well over a third of private hospital beds.[10] This creates conflicts of interest, with the state acting as funder of the public sector and regulator, and now investor, in the for-profit sector.

Malaysia has a young population, with the Economist Intelligence Unit (EIU) estimating that around half the population was under 25 in 2010. The proportion of over 65s is rising, however, and with it the incidence of long-term conditions such as hypertension and diabetes (up by 43 per cent and 88 per cent respectively between 2002 and 2012).[11] The EIU also notes that in the 15 years to 2011 the percentage of the population which was overweight or obese tripled from 5 per cent to 15 per cent.[12]

With a tropical climate, Malaysia suffers from the mosquito-borne dengue fever and malaria. In rural areas the training of volunteers to assist in malaria surveillance, community prevention programmes and the provision of basic primary care has helped achieve a substantial reduction in malaria infections.

Conclusion

While Malaysia procrastinates over its necessary health reforms, the private sector continues to invest both at home and abroad. A clear government-sponsored plan for health system development over the next decade would continue the country's impressive long-term story of health improvement and help all stakeholders and citizens look forward to healthier, happier lives.

References

1 Ministry of Health, 1Care for 1Malaysia: Restructuring the Malaysian Health System (Government of Malaysia, 2009).

2 World Bank statistics, Life expectancy at birth (World Bank, 1957 & 2013).

3 Department of Statistics, Vital statistics: infant mortality per 1,000 live births (Government of Malaysia, 2012).

4 World Bank statistics, Total health expenditure (% of GDP) (World Bank, 2012).

5 Rasiah R. et al., 'Markets and healthcare services in Malaysia,' *Institutions and Economies*, 3(3), 467–86.

6 Prospect Group, WHO Global Health Observatory, Life expectancy data by country (WHO, 2012).

7 Interview with the President of Private Hospitals Association of Malaysia (Prospect Website, 15 January 2013).

8 Ministry of Health Malaysia, 1Care for 1Malaysia: Concept paper (Government of Malaysia, 2009).

9 Malaysia Healthcare Travel Council, Industry Statistics (MHTC, 2014).

10 Chee-Khoon C., The Malaysian health system in transition: The ambiguity of public and private (Municipal Services Project, 2014).

11 Economist Intelligence Unit, How sustainable is Malaysian healthcare? (EIU, April 2014).

12 Economist Intelligence Unit, Industry report, Healthcare, Malaysia (EIU, April 2014), p. 13.

7 Singapore
Wealth and health

For centuries Singapore has occupied a strategically important position in Asian and world trade. This small country, with a population of just over five million and with no substantive natural resources, has grown to become a significant player in political, social and economic affairs throughout the region. Its drive to trade with other countries and unashamedly learn, adopt and adapt from them has seen its living standards rise dramatically since independence in 1965. Singapore has one of the highest proportions of millionaires in the world and its GDP per head is over US$56,000.[1]

The economic growth generated by many of Asia's economies in recent decades has pulled millions from poverty into a new middle class that is demanding more and better services from their governments. Increasingly affluent citizens want public pensions, national health insurance, unemployment benefits and other hallmarks of social protection. Whether it is the ruling elite in China or the dominant People's Action Party (PAP) in Singapore, politicians in Asia realise they must deliver social reform and expand benefits or suffer lost support and even civil disorder.

They also realise, however, that it would be a mistake to make unfunded promises to be paid for by future generations and they have little desire to replace Asian traditions of hard work and thrift with a culture of welfare dependency. While the West boasts the welfare state accomplishments of Bismarck and Beveridge in the nineteenth and twentieth centuries, countries such as Singapore seek a more affordable balance between individual entitlement and social responsibility for the twenty-first century.

Singapore boasts one of the best health systems in the world and one of the highest life expectancies, standing at 82.3 years.[2] Infant mortality is just 2.7 per 1,000 live births.[3] Remarkably, it only spends 4.6 per cent of its GDP on health[4] – a figure virtually unchanged since independence – while promoting itself as a world-class centre for healthcare, clinical research, and biomedical and life science industries. As the country was being established, politicians and officials in Singapore looked at health and welfare systems around the world and were able to design one based on a blending of personal responsibility and social solidarity. Consequently, Singapore offers universal healthcare but the country's mixed financing delivery system requires patients to pay a substantial proportion of the cost; barely a third of total health expenditure currently comes from the state.[5]

3Ms

There are three government-operated funding schemes, known as the 3Ms: Medisave, MediShield and Medifund. Medisave is a straightforward savings scheme enabling citizens to put aside money for their and their families' healthcare expenses. MediShield is a low-cost insurance scheme; premiums can be paid out of Medisave accounts because it is intended that patients can buy this additional cover if their Medisave funds are insufficient. Medifund is a safety net for those who cannot afford their part of subsidised healthcare expenses. But a striking feature of the system is that there is little risk pooling; this can leave individuals who fall into serious ill health facing catastrophic costs. Singapore has a high level of income inequality and the overriding emphasis on personal payment of medical expenses exacerbates this divide. Some have questioned whether the 3M system truly provides universal healthcare. This has been the troubling reality beneath the overall impressive performance of the country's healthcare system.

However, there should be some improvement with the replacement of MediShield with a new scheme, MediShield Life, approved by Parliament in January 2015. It is a significant enhancement over the existing scheme, providing better protection against large hospital bills and expensive chronic treatments. Claim limits are being increased while co-insurance rates (where the insured person covers a set percentage of the covered costs after the deductible has been paid) are being cut from 10–20 per cent to 3–10 per cent. Under the new system, the lifetime claim limit is removed and the limit on annual claims increased; there are also increased daily limits for hospital stays and increases for surgical outpatient and cancer treatment limits. Premiums will increase, but subsidies should help many Singaporeans in the first few years.

Hospital wards are graded according to their facilities: the greater the state subsidy, the lower the grade of facilities. According to government figures, around three-quarters of admissions are to public hospitals, while just 20 per cent of primary healthcare is provided by the public sector.[6]

Electoral Shock

The ability of Singapore to plan for the future is impressive, but it needs to do more. The government is aware that the ageing population and an increase in Western-style chronic diseases mean its low GDP spend on health cannot continue. In the 2011 election, PAP was shocked to receive its lowest share of the vote since independence. It realised it needed to get closer to the hopes and fears of its citizens. While immigration was a key election issue, healthcare also figured prominently and this has prompted a series of announcements by the Ministry of Health. Its Healthcare 2020 master plan has three strategic objectives: enhance accessibility, improve quality and ensure the affordability of healthcare for Singaporeans.

Government spending on healthcare is starting to rise sharply. A rise of 22 per cent was forecast between 2013/14 and 2014/15 (from SG$5.8bn to SG$7.1bn).[7] These increases will expand both capacity and infrastructure as well as improve pay to cope with a looming workforce crisis. General hospitals and community hospitals are being built, along with additional primary care facilities. Specialised centres of excellence for treating heart disease, eye diseases and cancer, among other illnesses, are being built close to the general hospitals for better integration and accessibility. It is envisaged that by 2020 public hospital beds will increase by 30 per cent while community hospital beds will double, as will long-term care services, nursing homes, and domiciliary care and rehabilitation facilities.

Clinical training and development will be expanded and a third medical school – a joint venture between Singapore's Nanyang Technological University and Imperial College, London – started admitting students in 2013. Substantial pay rises for doctors and other healthcare professionals are part of a plan to recruit an additional 20,000 healthcare staff by 2020. This could fuel health pay across the region.

Singapore's population is ageing fast; it is estimated that, by 2030, 20 per cent of the population will be over 65.[8] To meet the challenges faced by many Asian countries with ageing populations and falling fertility rates, Singapore has introduced ElderShield, an insurance scheme to cover the costs of private nursing homes and other expenses in old age. Introduced in 2002, it has over one million policy holders already,[9] and the government is set to make enhancements to the scheme. Referring to the founding of the state, the government has cleverly justified this investment by describing the baby boomers now reaching old age as the Pioneer Generation.

The approach of the Singapore government to healthcare has often been described as 'steering rather than rowing', and this can be seen in its approach to prevention. It is estimated that by 2020 roughly 85 per cent of people aged over 65 years will be healthy and reasonably active,[10] and the government is aggressively pushing people to stay healthy with screening and healthy lifestyle programmes – including free exercise programmes in the central business district – along with more community support. It takes a similarly robust approach to keeping children close to their ideal weight, with programmes supporting those who are overweight or underweight. Only 14 per cent of the population smokes, one of the lowest rates in Asia.[11]

In 2009 the Ministry of Health established the Agency for Integrated Care to improve integration across the care sectors. The aim was to address concerns that while the government has invested heavily in hospitals, people with chronic conditions are struggling to get the right care in the community, whether in their own home or in a nursing home. Regional health systems (a strange term for a city state) are being established to link general hospitals with community rehabilitation centres and primary and community care. However, the strategy for integration relies on unequal forces collaborating. Partly as a show of national strength, Singapore has always invested heavily in hospitals, which have become isolated from other services. Hospital medical staff hold huge power while fragmented family and community practitioners play second fiddle in a system that revolves around secondary and tertiary care. This is getting better but more pace needs to be put into the reforms.

Exploiting Technology

Integration will be encouraged by further development of the National Electronic Health Record programme. Launched in 2011, it is already used by more than 280 institutions.[12] Telehealth and telemedicine are increasingly being deployed, for example to support stroke rehabilitation at home and to allow hospital ophthalmologists to give patients in polyclinics virtual eye examinations.

Singapore's biomedical science industry and medical research are world class, and its clinical research, trials and commercialisation – all supported by strong intellectual property protection and exacting industry standards – continue to expand. State support is substantial, for example the Biomedical Science Industry Partnership Office helps businesses join forces with multiple Singaporean agencies charged with growing health and wealth.

The government is keen to promote Singapore as a primary destination for medical tourism and the well-developed private sector has plans to expand hospital capacity to cater for a large influx of foreign patients. In an attempt to reduce public waiting times, the government also anticipates using spare private sector capacity; from 2015, private health provider Raffles Medical Group will start receiving non-critical ambulance cases at costs similar to public hospitals.

Conclusion

Singapore has a plan for its healthcare reforms, the perseverance to push on with them and the resources to finance them. But patients' needs are changing: the population is ageing quickly and the dominance of private over state funding means not everyone has access to the care they need. It is not yet clear if the country is willing to reform its care system quickly enough to keep pace. If its plan to strengthen primary and community care and integrate care more effectively is to work, the government needs to be more radical in taking on vested interests. It is clear from talking to senior officials that this urgency is appreciated but not yet fully grasped. The inequity of the emphasis on personal funding also remains a concern, although the MediShield Life development is a welcome move.

Singapore could spend a lot of money over the next five years propping up twentieth-century models of care and hiking pay to levels which cause problems across the region. Alternatively, it could map out an exciting future enabled by technology and shift to new channels which will enhance this country's enviable reputation for innovation and progress.

References

1 World Bank statistics, GDP per capita (World Bank, 2014).

2 World Bank statistics, Life expectancy at birth (World Bank, 2013).

3 World Bank statistics, Infant mortality rate (per 1,000 live births) (World Bank, 2013).

4 World Bank statistics, Total health expenditure (% of GDP), (World Bank, 2013).

5 World Bank statistics, Public health expenditure (% of total health expenditure) (World Bank, 2012).

6 Ministry of Health, Health Institution Statistics: Introduction to Healthcare Institution Statistics (MOH Singapore, 2012).

7 Economist Intelligence Unit, Healthcare Report: Singapore (EIU, 2014).

8 Wen et al., 'Futures of Ageing in Singapore,' *Journal of Futures Studies*, 17(3), 81–102 (2013).

9 Economist Intelligence Unit, Healthcare Report: Singapore (EIU, 2014).

10 Haseline W.A., *Affordable Excellence: The Singapore Health Story* (Brookings Institution Press, 2013), p. 131.

11 Ministry of Health statistics, Daily smoking prevalence among adults (MOH Singapore, 2012).

12 Khalik S, Minister lauds ways IT benefits patients (Singapore Silver Pages, 16 September 2014).

8 Indonesia

Largest single payer in the world

I first encountered Indonesia's breath taking beauty as a tourist in 1992. I toured a then-underdeveloped Bali, Lombok and a few of the Gili Islands. The Indonesian archipelago boasts over 18,000 small islands, of which fewer than half have been named and under a thousand permanently inhabited. It is a nation of many contrasts, not only in geography but between wealth and poverty, and has almost unrivalled ambition for its healthcare.

In many respects, Indonesia is on the up. Economic growth is good (between 5.2 per cent and 6.5 per cent over the last five years)[1] and it is beginning to take its place on the global stage as the world's fourth most populous country (250 million people) and third-largest democracy.

Incredibly, for those accustomed to the ageing West, 29 per cent of the population is under 15 and only 5 per cent of the population is 65 or over.[2] This young demographic profile presents both challenges and opportunities for President Joko Widodo. For example, it has been suggested that over one-third of children under five have stunted growth.[3] Besides having high personal costs such as chronic disease and delayed cognitive development, stunting and malnutrition undermine the economy. UNICEF estimates that the country could be losing out on 2 per cent to 3 per cent of growth every year as a result of poor productivity and underachieving human capital.

That said, Indonesia has become something of a poster boy for improving prosperity and is certainly considered a darling among emerging markets, with over a decade of sustained growth. Its master plan – the Acceleration and Expansion for Indonesia's Economic Development 2011–25 – calls for sustainable policies that are pro-growth, pro-jobs, pro-poor and pro-green. Action is coordinated across the policy spectrum, with investment in financial services, infrastructure, education, eco-friendly tourism, community development and health to name but a few. All intended to create a virtuous circle of improvement and self-supporting sustainability. It is in this light that Indonesia's audacious aspirations for universal healthcare should be viewed and applauded.

Big Ambitions

Currently, Indonesia spends 3.1 per cent of GDP on health[4] and has an average life expectancy of 70.8 years.[5] It spends less on its healthcare than its neighbours Thailand, Vietnam and the Philippines and its public health system has suffered years of underinvestment, even though health was a priority under the 10-year rule of Susilo Bambang Yudhoyono.[6] In January 2014, the Jaminan Kesehatan Nasional (JKN, or National Health Insurance) was launched with the unambiguous intention of providing universal health insurance by 2019. This makes it the largest single-payer health insurance scheme in the world.

Initially concentrating on integrating a number of existing schemes, mainly for the poor, the Economist Intelligence Unit forecasts that health spending will increase by 12 per cent per year to a total of US$46 billion by 2018–19.[7] This means increased health spending per head from US$102 in 2014 to US$177. With further commitments in recent months, those figures could rise even faster. The scale and reach of the JKN is enormous: it is estimated that it will cover 122 million people (nearly twice the population of the UK) in its first year. In a hopeful sign of things to come, the government has doubled the size of the budget and incorporated 86 million people from one of the existing schemes, Jamkesmas.[8] Membership of the new scheme will increase further as wage earners in the formal sector contribute 5 per cent of their salary and other members begin to pay monthly premiums. It is hoped that by widening coverage the risk pool will be strong enough to support development.

Similar schemes have been considered in nearby Malaysia but many employers were anxious that funds would be poorly used or result in compromised economic competitiveness. The Indonesian government is more resolute, with a broad plan and sound economic justification for strengthening universal healthcare, arguing that it will boost productivity and competitiveness. That said, during my most recent visit there was growing concern that the absence of a clear, long-term financial plan for universal healthcare could undermine confidence.

One of the architects of the new scheme, Professor Hasbullah Thabrany from Universitas Indonesia, believes the scheme has momentum.[9] He said: 'The good thing is that the JKN programme has started. To use a metaphor of a car – the engine has started but there are a number of problems, because the fuel is not right.' He was referring to the funding: he is concerned that the amount the government is paying for healthcare for the poor is well below market cost, which may force providers to compromise quality or not participate in the programme.

In my experience, developing a comprehensive universal healthcare insurance system in little over five years is unprecedented, but the total scope depends on the breadth and depth of coverage. Some schemes for other low- to middle-earning countries concentrate on preventative, primary and community care.

In this sense, cover can be broad but not deep and access to secondary and tertiary care is limited. It is not surprising that Indonesia has looked carefully at developments in Mexico and Brazil, where such approaches have been pursued with considerable success.

In Indonesia there are problems with the supply side. The number of hospital beds is one of the lowest in Asia at 0.9 per 1,000 people,[10] and is heavily skewed to cities such as Jakarta. Mirroring this, the number of doctors is 0.3 per 1,000[11] and too many practise in towns and cities. There are incentives to practise in rural areas, but more needs to be done if healthcare is to take root everywhere. While the national average bed ratio has doubled in the last few years, in some regions it fell sharply due to tight budgets and a poorly executed attempt to decentralise power to districts.

Some doctors have complained about the workload and rates of reimbursement associated with the introduction of the JKN. Dr Damroh at Bekasi General Hospital in Jakarta says that since the JKN was implemented the number of patients coming to them has doubled: 'Now, we get an average 1,000 patients per day and 800 of these are JKN patients.'[12]

According to some, this pressure is exactly what is needed to spur investment. Financial services leviathan Standard Chartered says: 'We expect the JKN roll-out to drive demand for inpatient and outpatient services at public hospitals and participating private hospitals, as large ticket hospitalisation and specialist expenses will be covered by JKN. We estimate overall hospital services markets will increase at a 2013–23 [compound annual growth rate] of 13–16%.'[13] It estimates JKN members already have access to more than 9,000 community clinics and 1,700 out of Indonesia's 2,300 hospitals.

Indonesia's growing middle class is providing a market for healthcare services overseas in countries such as Singapore. Around 1.5 million Indonesians currently travel overseas for healthcare, costing the country an estimated US$1.4bn a year[14] in lost potential revenue for the country's own private sector.

Indonesia's already huge population continues to grow at around 1.2 per cent,[15] or around 3 million extra human beings, every year. Even for an established health service, keeping pace with such population growth would be hard. Its need to increase the numbers of doctors, nurses and midwives rapidly is making it difficult to control medical education standards and staff quality. Once they are qualified, the poor pay for public sector staff means doctors often run private clinics as well as work in the public sector, making absenteeism in public primary care clinics a cause for concern.

The sheer size of Indonesia and the remoteness of many areas are serious impediments to universal healthcare. The distribution of doctors, nurses, midwives, beds, equipment and medical supplies will always be a big challenge. The government hopes technology such as online consultations will help, but this can only be a partial solution.

The Burden of Disease

More than 28 million Indonesians live below the poverty line, and roughly half of all households remain clustered around it – set at just under US$17 a month.[16] Infectious diseases such as malaria, dengue fever and tuberculosis are a serious problem, particularly in the remote eastern regions. In 2011, polio and measles outbreaks among children prompted a mass immunisation programme.

Indonesia, Pakistan and the Philippines are the only three countries in Asia with rising HIV/AIDS infection rates[17]; WHO estimates that around 640,000 Indonesians are living with HIV/AIDS,[18] with only 6 per cent receiving antiretroviral drugs.[19] Public education is hampered by religious sensitivities which make it difficult to discuss issues such as homosexuality or extramarital relationships.

The rate of smoking is awful: more than two-thirds of Indonesian men smoke and 400,000 Indonesians die every year from smoking-related illnesses.[20] Although malnutrition is a bigger problem than obesity, diabetes is thought to be increasing at around 6 per cent a year. If this continues, by 2030 almost 12 million Indonesians will have the disease.[21] A significant proportion of Indonesians still do not have access to sanitation. Maternal mortality remains high.

It seems to me that the success of universal healthcare in Indonesia relies on timing, speed, momentum, confidence and upfront investment. In many developing countries, health policy experts rhetorically ask 'what comes first, the health plan or the doctors?', implying that universal coverage can only proceed as fast as the supply of healthcare infrastructure and staff and vice versa. While this is always true up to a point, articulating a vision, having a plan and creating momentum are some of the best ways governments can make quick and lasting improvements to health status. Being professional and transparent in the way the plan is executed are also important.

While around three-quarters of hospitals are in the public sector, the enthusiasm of some private sector players is crucial for sustainable development. In discussions with private sector health organisations in Indonesia, I noticed some emerging trends. The first, epitomised by leading private healthcare provider Siloam, is to provide services to the JKN under the same roof as its private facilities. Siloam plans to build around 40 hospitals by 2017, almost tripling its number of beds to around 10,000. I have seen how some of its private facilities are co-located with public ones providing decent standards of care to the general population.

The second trend is the private sector embracing universal healthcare but thinking that the inevitable overcrowding of public hospitals through improved access will encourage the aspiring and middle classes to seek private facilities. Some forecasts suggest that Indonesia's middle and affluent classes will double between 2013 and 2020 from 74 million to 144 million people.[22] Some operators will focus exclusively on this cohort and look to expand in second-tier cities (as is happening in India).

Private sector players from outside healthcare are also interested in making long-term investments. I met executives from some of the property development groups which have announced plans to expand their hospital business beyond Jakarta and explore whether new housing developments should incorporate community and hospital facilities. One of their key concerns was the availability of high-quality medical and nursing staff, particularly now that the Indonesian medical authorities have restricted the arrival of foreign doctors. This policy, driven by protectionism among doctors, blocks one of the major options for addressing the serious shortage of medical staff. The current plan to address the crisis by accelerating the number of graduates looks overly ambitious.

The growing role of the private sector in healthcare raises questions about access for the wider population. There are laws requiring private operators to provide subsidised services to the poor but there are many incidents of significant out-of-pocket charges being levied.

Conclusion

As Indonesia pursues its ambition of establishing the world's largest single-payer health system it has one unusual advantage in that President Widodo has first-hand experience of implementing a health insurance system, having created a similar one in Jakarta when he was governor. The size of the population, the remoteness of many areas, the endemic poverty and the high burden of disease mean it will take many years to establish universal healthcare, but their ambition is laudable. If they continue on the path to reform, they will give other low-income countries hope. As always, financial and political stability will be crucial to long-term success.

References

1 World Bank, Economic growth figures (World Bank, 2010–2015).

2 World Bank, Population age figures (World Bank, 2013).

3 Economist Intelligence Unit, Indonesia economy: Public-health challenges under Jokowi, (EIU, November 2014).

4 World Bank statistics, Total health expenditure (% of GDP) (World Bank, 2013).

5 World Bank statistics, Life expectancy at birth (World Bank, 2013).

6 Economist Intelligence Unit, Industry Report, Healthcare (EIU, December 2014), p. 4.

7 EIU (2014).

8 Das R., Emerald of the equator: Indonesia the next healthcare frontier (Forbes, 29 December 2014).

9 Wirdana A., Inadequate funding may hamper Indonesia health insurance scheme (The Establishment Post, 10 November 2014).

10 World Bank, Hospital beds (per 1,000 people) (World Bank, 2012).

11 OECD, OECD Health Statistics 2014. How does Indonesia compare? (2014), p. 2.

12 Wirdana A., Inadequate funding may hamper Indonesia health insurance scheme (The Establishment Post, 10 November 2014).

13 Standard Chartered, Equity research briefing – Indonesia healthcare: The power of healing (Standard Chartered, 2014), p. 5.

14. Chiong L.W., Big gaps in Indonesia healthcare (*The Business Times*, 10 August 2012).

15 World Bank, Population growth (annual %) (World Bank, 2012).

16 Indonesia overview, The World Bank (October 2014).

17 EIU (2014), p.12.

18 World Health Organization, Number of people (all ages) living with HIV (WHO, 2013).

19 World Health Organization, Estimated antiretroviral therapy coverage among people living with HIV (%) (WHO, 2013).

20 EIU (2014), p.13.

21 International Diabetes Federation, Diabetes Atlas 6th ed. (IDF, 2013), p. 160.

22 Rastogi V. et al., BCG Perspectives: Indonesia's rising middle class and affluent consumers (Boston Consulting Group, 2013).

9 Australia
Advance Australia Fair

I have loved Australia ever since I worked in Melbourne and Sydney during my time on the NHS Management Training Scheme in 1991. It is a country full of hope and optimism, whose expanding and increasingly mixed population reflects how it is capitalising on the growth of Asia. Every week the population increases by 8,000 people, half of which seek to live in the cosmopolitan cities of Sydney and Melbourne.[1] Australia now has a population in excess of 23 million people and difficult trade-offs between health, infrastructure and other public expenditure are being made to tackle its debts. On my recent trips, I have seen how the demographic, social, political and economic changes since I first worked there have influenced the development of its health economy.

Back in 1991, the health service in Australia was one of the finest in the world. Today, it is still ranked fourth by the Commonwealth Fund but it has not developed as quickly as it might have.[2] The reform and rejuvenation process has been thwarted by the political blame game between the federal and state governments. Unlike Canada, which delegates nearly all health control to the provinces, Australia broadly has federal authorities running primary care and the states running hospital care. This, coupled with the country's fractious politics, has held back reforms needed to make care models fit for future needs, especially the demands of chronic disease and ageing.

That said, Australian healthcare has many strengths. With a GDP health spend around the OECD average of 9.4 per cent,[3] life expectancy is high at 82.2 years[4] and clinical outcomes are good. There has been a substantial reduction in deaths from heart attack and other circulatory diseases and Australia can boast one of the lowest smoking rates in the world (16 per cent, down from 34 per cent in 1983[5]).

One of the key characteristics of Australia's health system is its plurality – public and private sectors play a major role in both the funding and provision of care, under a common national framework. The publicly funded system, Medicare, was established in 1984 with the aim of providing 'the most equitable and efficient means of providing health insurance coverage for all Australians'.[6] At heart, Medicare has always been a funding system rather than a provider, and has three main components: the Medicare Benefits Schedule (offering subsidised non-hospital care), the Pharmaceutical Benefits Scheme (subsidising drug costs) and free access to most hospital care for those who elect to be public patients. Medicare is funded through a hypothecated 2 per cent income tax, with the balance met by general taxation.

The Balance of Public and Private Funding

Over the decades there has been a great deal of policy experimentation exploring the right balance between public and private funding. Recent governments have encouraged people to take out private health insurance in an attempt to contain Medicare costs. On one level this has been successful: around 55 per cent of Australians now have some form of private health cover (up from 30 per cent in the 1990s). However, costs continue to rise sharply, with Medicare expenditure forecast to increase from A$19 billion in 2013–14 to A$23.6 billion in 2016–17.[7] Overall, the government now accounts for around 67 per cent of healthcare spending, markedly lower than the OECD average of 72 per cent.

Australia's provider sector is similarly mixed. Private hospitals now account for about one-third of beds (half for-profit, half not-for-profit) and are responsible for two-thirds of elective care. This approach has produced a good elective care system, with acceptable waiting times and decent choice between public and private hospitals. However, weak integration between emergency, community and primary care services is causing problems in emergency departments. Some states, such as New South Wales, are exploring the benefits of greater collaboration between hospitals and primary care: New South Wales' Integrated Care Programme is incentivising various collaborative models between Local Health Districts, primary care organisations and GPs.

Barriers to Change

The mixed system of funding and provision pursued by Australia has added much-needed capacity and kept quality high. However, a fragmented distribution of power and control has created one of the system's most enduring barriers to change. Australia suffers from the 'triple whammy' of separate financing streams (federal and state), separate funding streams (primary and secondary) and separate employment relationships (some doctors and the rest of hospital staff). This makes large-scale reform difficult. As the burden of disease shifts towards chronic diseases, pressure points have exposed the need for a more coordinated approach across these various funding and service provision streams. Care integration is becoming more and more urgent in terms of both care quality and system sustainability but the status quo is proving hard to shift. A case in point is payment systems, which are prevented from moving away from episodic (and, for most primary care physicians, fee-for-service) reimbursement to value-based contracting by powerful defences of the status quo, especially by the medical establishment.

One of the most serious attempts to reform the health system came under the Rudd/Gillard administrations in 2007–13. In 2008, the National Health and

Hospitals Reform Commission was established to address many deep-seated issues. With an ambitious 123 recommendations, the commission sought to reform both financing and delivery. The supreme decision-making body representing all states and territories, the Council of Australian Governments (COAG), agreed that the federal government would assume responsibility for primary care and take majority funding responsibility for public hospitals, paying a 60 per cent share of the cost using an efficient activity-based funding approach. Governance was to be strengthened through greater devolution to aggregated hospital boards, improved efficiency through a new Independent Hospital Pricing Authority, and transparency through a National Health Performance Authority. Medicare Locals were established to support preventative action in local communities and better coordinate care for chronic diseases; these have now been superseded in 2015 by Primary Health Networks.

At the time, these recommendations were broadly endorsed but, as the new right-leaning coalition assumed power in 2014, the Chairman of the COAG Reform Council reported on the healthcare system after five years of reform.[8] Progress had been made in life expectancy and infant mortality and access to primary care, alongside a small improvement in emergency services, but waiting times for elective surgery had increased slightly and older people had to wait longer to get residential care. So the report showed progress but it was patchy and limited. The changes did not have sufficient time nor the momentum to encourage greater collaboration between federal and state levels or between hospitals, primary care and community services.

In the 2014 general election the most important issues were the economy and debt. The new government acted swiftly and reversed many of the reforms, arguing that the cost had not produced sufficient benefits for patients or taxpayers. The Budget for Health published in May 2014 prioritised action to kick-start the economy and reduce debt 'to build a strong, prosperous economy and safe, secure Australia'.[9] Citizens were expected to make a greater contribution to the cost of their own care. Billions of dollars were to be taken from budgets, including the termination of a state-level preventative health programme. A A$7 co-payment for GP consultations was proposed, along with cuts to the Medicare safety net, but both were defeated by the Senate following a public backlash.

Defending its decisions, the Coalition pointed to the dramatic and unaffordable increase in healthcare costs, highlighting that over the previous 11 years health expenditure increases were greater than the combined growth of all other major areas of government spending. As politicians frequently remind us, 'to govern is to choose' and the Coalition prioritised debt reduction and a stronger economy, hoping these will, in time, produce the growth needed to fund healthcare. But money alone will not solve the deep-seated issues that become more pressing every day as the population both grows and ages. Structural problems and fragmented care remain prominent features, and demand and supply pressures continue apace.

Reforms in the States and Territories

Future funding settlements between the federal and state level are now part of a major review by COAG – the Reform of the Federation – that will recommend policy on the roles, responsibilities and contributions of the states and territories and the federal government. The federal government has signalled its intent to cap its contributions to states for public hospitals from 2017/18 thereby creating a looming 'fiscal cliff' that will signal further productivity improvements and efficiency gains.

In the meantime, individual states are attempting their own, more limited, paths towards reform. Queensland is moving to a greater public–private mix, with Western Australia pushing in a similar direction. New South Wales is exploring the benefits of greater collaboration between hospitals. Tasmania is well suited to greater primary and secondary care integration and could be a test bed for new care pathways. South Australia will continue to strengthen primary care, mental health and hospital services and the Northern Territories will continue their good work on Aboriginal health, community services and devolved accountability frameworks.

Its fractious politics aside, Australia is a magnificent place to live. It ranked first on the 2014 OECD Better Life Index, which measures social determinants that support good mental health such as employment, civic participation, education, sense of community and work–life balance. It is an attractive place for clinicians, and over the last decade hundreds of doctors have left Europe for Australia; the pay is better, hours are shorter, jobs are often easier to find and the lifestyle is appealing. Clinicians are generally regarded as having less bureaucracy to cope with and more freedom, although that doesn't necessarily translate into better care.

Progressive Mental Health

One of the most notable features of Australia's healthcare system is its progressive approach to mental health. In moving away from the old model of 'warehousing' psychiatric patients in hospitals, it has developed a proactive community system with many services, such as crisis and home treatment, early intervention and assertive outreach based on a life-course approach.

Access to psychological services has been increased through the Better Access Initiative. Other services include the Personal Helpers and Mentors programme and the Support for Day to Day Living in the Community programme. Police training in working with people suffering from mental illness has been improved and Australian developers have been behind a number of highly innovative mobile- and computer-based interventions to improve mental health.

But there is still room for improvement in mental health services, with the mix of federal and state funding and public, private and voluntary sector provision making services fragmented and complex. A National Mental Health Commission has been reviewing the whole system with the aim of creating a more integrated approach, with a stronger focus on supporting recovery. The commission is concerned about mental health among Aboriginal and Torres Strait Islander peoples; the suicide rate is roughly double the figure for other Australians.

Indigenous Australians

While there have been improvements in health services and outcomes for indigenous Australians (most notably immunisation rates), serious disparities remain, with life expectancy for these communities on average 10 years shorter than for the rest of the population.[10] Between 1997 and 2010 there was a 24 per cent fall in the number of Aboriginal and Torres Strait Islander people who died from avoidable causes – a remarkable achievement – yet still twice as many infants are born with a low birth weight compared with non-indigenous infants.[11] Indigenous peoples make up around 3 per cent of the population but account for less than 1 per cent of the healthcare workforce.[12] All Aboriginal and Torres Strait Islander people are entitled to an annual health check designed for indigenous people, but in 2013–14 fewer than one in four attended. While access to care in remote areas remains an issue, the poor health outcomes are mostly driven by continuing socio-economic disadvantages, such as poor access to education, low incomes, overcrowded housing and poor nutrition.

Despite its sporty image, one of the biggest risks facing Australian healthcare is obesity; it has the fifth highest rate in the OECD, behind the United States, Mexico, New Zealand and Hungary.[13] According to the OECD more than a third of Australians aged over 15 are overweight and almost the same number again are obese. Around 57 per cent of Australians do not do enough exercise and chronic disease is now the leading cause of illness and disability, accounting for around 90 per cent of all deaths.[14]

Conclusion

Australia will always be a magnificent country to live in but it must be more ambitious for its health services if they wish to remain both sustainable and high quality in the long term. It provides excellent healthcare to most of its citizens but care service design and system reform need to keep pace.

While the economic situation means that states are rightly prioritising the financial pressures they face, healthcare reform needs to be recognised as a means of achieving these goals and not seen as a luxury or distraction. National direction has largely been abandoned in favour of state and regional experimentation, and the status quo continues to be locked in by the triple whammy of separate financing, funding and employment streams. Australians are increasing in number, increasing in age and increasing in morbidity. The time to act is now.

References

1 *The Australian*, Healthcare and infrastructure spend tearing budget apart (*The Australian*, 6 May 2014).

2 Commonwealth Fund, Mirror on the wall: How the performance of the US healthcare system performs internationally – 2014 Update (Commonwealth Fund: New York, 2014).

3 World Bank statistics, Total health expenditure (% of GDP) (World Bank, 2013).

4 World Bank statistics, Life expectancy at birth (World Bank, 2013).

5 OECD, Health statistics 2014: How does Australia compare? (OECD, 2014).

6 From a speech by Minister for Social Security Bill Hayden on second reading of the Health Insurance Bill 1973 (29 November 1973).

7 Australian Government, Budget Strategy and Outlook: 2013–14 (Australian Government, 2013).

8 COAG Reform Council, Healthcare in Australia 2012–13: Five years of performance (Australian Government, 2014).

9 Commonwealth of Australia, Budget: Health 2014/15 (Australian Government, 2014).

10 Australian Institute for Health and Welfare, Mortality and life expectancy of Indigenous Australians 2008 to 2012 (AIHW, 2014).

11 Department of Health and Ageing, Aboriginal and Torres Strait Islander Health Performance Framework (Australian Government, 2012).

12 Australian Institute of Health and Welfare, The health and welfare of Australia's Aboriginal and Torres Strait Islander people: An overview (Australian Government, 2011).

13 OECD, OECD health statistics 2014: How does Australia compare? (OECD, 2014).

14 Australian Institute for Health and Welfare, Australia's Health 2014 (Australian Government, 2014).

10 India
One country, two worlds

To work in Indian healthcare is truly to see some of the best and worst of what the world's systems have to offer.

Private chains of healthcare providers in India are innovating with a speed and scale that shatters the myth that only wealthy countries can afford high-quality care. By combining American assembly line methods, Japanese lean management techniques and a uniquely Indian 'jugaad' (a Hindi word meaning to solve complex problems with ingeniously simple solutions), these organisations are able to offer Western levels of quality at at a fraction of the cost.

Narayana Health, for example, is a chain of 26 multi-speciality hospitals that exploit economies of scale at every opportunity to improve quality and reduce cost. Its largest facility is a 5,000-bed 'health city': a factory for cardiac surgery and cancer care with the fixed costs spread across as many patients as possible. It further leverages scale by centralising support services across the network – teleradiology is done in a single hub in Bangalore and purchasing is unified across the chain. With 15 per cent of India's market for cardiac surgery, Narayana creates its own suppliers if it feels it could be paying less for products, such as when it reduced the price paid for surgical gowns from US$100 to US$12 per operation by guaranteeing a group of business graduates a sole-supplier deal if they could create a product that did the same job for less.

Where centralisation is less achievable – for example when trying to improve access outside of major cities – Narayana is single-minded in cutting out costs wherever they don't add value to patient care. It recently completed its first low-cost facility, a 300-bed cardiac hospital built in six months at a cost of US$6 million. Ultimately, Narayana's audacious goal is to perform heart operations at a cost of US$800 per patient. I toured facilities with Dr Devi Shetty, chairman and founder of Narayana, and have no doubt of his conviction and ability to transform care.

Two other world-leading private providers – Apollo Hospital and Aravind Eye Care – follow a similar model of using volume to increase quality while decreasing cost. A major part of the formula is leveraging the scarce professional skills of doctors to the maximum degree possible: they only work on tasks that require a doctor, with other activities like pre- and post-operative care delegated to task-specialist support workers. Aravind doctors perform 1,000 to 1,400 eye surgeries a year compared with an average of 400 among US doctors.[1] This is achieved by making sure doctors only do what only doctors can do.

Technology – another scarce resource – is also leveraged to its maximum capacity, such as in Apollo where scanners are run round the clock, with cheaper prices during less sociable hours. Both Aravind and Apollo stratify their pricing structure for patients so that the wealthy cross-subsidise the poor – again allowing volumes to increase and prices for those that do pay to be lower.

Many expected this production line method to result in worse outcomes, but both Aravind and Apollo demonstrate equivalent (and in some cases better) outcomes than is typical in the West because of the close relationship between volume and quality in surgery – the more someone does a procedure, the better they are at it.[2]

The Burden of Catastrophic Costs

Sadly, these islands of excellence are far from the norm. Of India's 1.2 billion population, only around 300 million have any kind of health insurance,[3] and those services which are accessible are often of dubious quality. This leaves India with a very high rate of catastrophic health expenditure – 18 per cent of all households.[4] The government has said that almost all hospitalisation episodes, even in public hospitals, lead to catastrophic expenditures. Around 63 million people every year face poverty because of healthcare costs, making it the leading cause of families falling back below the poverty line.[5]

The situation for most Indians is so bad that to even discuss hospitals may seem to some premature. Access to clean water, sanitation and an adequate diet are all tragically low. Half of the nation's children are malnourished[6] (50 per cent of all the malnourished children in the world) and 5 per cent die before their fifth birthday.[7] Many of these deaths are due to diarrhoeal diseases that would be survivable with rehydration salts costing less than US$1. Only a third of the population (36 per cent) have access to adequate sanitation.[8] So, as exciting as the new hyper-efficient hospital chains coming out of India are, the most dramatic improvements to life expectancy will be achieved through basics such as food, toilets and vaccinations.

India spends very little on healthcare – just 4 per cent of GDP, or US$61 per person per year. This compares with US$322 in China, US$887 in Russia and US$1,056 in Brazil.[9] The government's share of this expenditure is also very small – just 4 per cent of the Indian government's budget goes on health (1 per cent of total GDP).[10] With figures like these it is unsurprising that India has one of the world's highest rates of out-of-pocket expenditure for health.

These limited resources are deployed unevenly. Incredibly, just 2 per cent of India's doctors operate in rural areas, despite 68 per cent of the population living there.[11] There are large and ever-growing inequalities in health between regions. States such as Kerala have an infant mortality rate of 12 per 1,000 live births while in the rural state of Assam it is 56 per 1,000.[12]

A two-tier health service is now increasingly in effect and there is a very real danger of these parallel systems cementing themselves permanently. If the government does not act quickly, hundreds of millions will be left behind, creating a major drag on India's economic development and a serious source of future popular unrest.

The story of government health policy to date can be broadly summarised as encouraging private sector expansion in conjunction with well-designed but limited public health programmes. The National Rural Health Mission was established in 2005 and has developed a workforce of 900,000 community health volunteers and 178,000 new paid health workers.[13] The emphasis is primarily on reproductive health and control of specific priority diseases, with cash transfers and a fleet of 18,000 ambulances to try to improve access to the thinly scattered number of facilities that exist in rural areas. An equivalent programme for slum areas of cities – the National Urban Health Mission – started in 2013 with a similar approach of improving access to primary care and reproductive health through volunteers, community health workers, women's health committees and small primary care centres.

Meanwhile, the private sector has been booming with the help of state support. Eighty per cent of new beds built in India over the last decade are in for-profit facilities – mostly single-owner businesses of variable quality.[14] The government has created a fertile environment for this growth through generous tax exemptions and preferential allocation of land. The rapid growth of India's private healthcare sector is uncoordinated, however, and in recent visits to larger hospitals it is clear that there is overcapacity in many cities. With the recent liberalisation of the rules governing foreign investment in healthcare, a period of consolidation is on the horizon for India's private healthcare sector.

The good news is that under the government of Narendra Modi, India has its first serious national health plan in 13 years. The aim of the 2015 National Health Policy (NHP) is bold: to make healthcare a fundamental legal right and provide a basic level of primary, preventative and emergency coverage to the whole country by 2019. While much of the delivery of this goal will be devolved to state-level, the core features of the policy will be free access to drugs, diagnostics and emergency care, and an expansion of preventative programmes targeting nutrition, sanitation, traffic accidents and pollution. This said, the first Bharatiya Janata Party (BJP) budget did not offer the health funding and reform that many hoped for. Time will tell.

India needs a functioning universal health system if it is to fulfil its ambitions as a global economic powerhouse. The goals of the NHP are right, but it lacks a coherent approach as to how these will be achieved, especially in the role of the private sector which it both embraces (contracting out ambulatory services) and shuns (keeping primary care public). This may indicate a sophisticated mixing of the best of both worlds or, more probably, that the separate sections of the policy were created by separate teams within the Ministry of Health.

Mismanagement and Corruption

The cost of implementing the NHP has been estimated at US$26 billion over four years, a more-than-doubling in the share of public health expenditure (from 1 per cent of GDP to 2.5 per cent).[15] There was dismay, therefore, when just a few months after the NHP was announced, India's health budget was cut by 25 per cent. Though a disappointing sign, this highlights one of the biggest challenges facing India's efforts to achieve universal health coverage: even what little money is available often goes unspent. Mismanagement, bureaucracy and corruption are endemic at every level of the health system and act as a major barrier to money reaching its intended beneficiaries.[16] Experts refer to this as a lack of 'absorptive capacity' in the system, but in practical terms it means empty hospitals, overlapping programmes and underfunded services, with large budgetary surpluses at the end of each year. Many of the officials I have met are resigned to the dire quality of management in the public health system, or even find it amusing, but India will never make serious gains in coverage if failure is tolerated in this way.

I have some hope for the future of healthcare in India. Its pace and flair for frugal improvement has already benefited the world in so many ways, not least with its huge generics industry that has given us all cheaper pharmaceutical prices and was instrumental in breaking open access to antiretroviral drugs to millions of HIV-positive Africans, slowing the AIDS epidemic and saving countless lives. I strongly believe it can be a global cradle of innovation for healthcare delivery that will show the way in low-cost, high-quality services. The country has a huge opportunity to use its vast geography and young population as an asset by developing m-health and e-health at serious scale. If the protocol-based care of the private chains can be combined with its vast call centre sector and nascent medical device industry, India could not only achieve its goal of healthcare for all but also develop a major new export of cheap telemedicine and telecare to the world. The first signs of this are already emerging with maternal advice tools such as Dr Anita and pilots by Narayana to manage large volumes of patients with chronic conditions through telephone, email and text messaging.

Conclusion

India has the opportunity to become both a university and factory for the world's health workforce in the twenty-first century. The country itself needs an additional three million doctors over the next 20 years,[17] a requirement it will not achieve a fraction of with its current training model of Western-style professional education delivered by a collection of poorly equipped and traditional medical colleges. If it can instead leverage some of the more radical schemes to deliver Modi's goal of 'the world's most competitive workforce' it can redesign medical education with significant online and remote components and a far more targeted approach to the skills doctors will need for their particular speciality. Cutting the time and cost of training doctors would not only help India fill the enormous gaps in its healthcare workforce, but could transform it into a global exporter of healthcare talent, blending the precision of Western medical education with Eastern values of dignity and respect.

From its current position, these ideas may seem absurd, but the pace of social and economic change in the world's largest democracy is staggering. I was in Delhi on the day the BJP was swept out of power in the state by the two-year-old Aam Aadmi Party (AAP, or Common Man's Party). The biggest landslide in the state's electoral history was driven by a popular movement demanding cheaper electricity, better access to water and the tackling of corruption.

So far, for reasons that are unclear to me, people in India for the most part tolerate poor-quality or no healthcare. Perhaps they are hoping that the rising tide of the economic middle class will eventually reach them, but progress will not be fast enough for most, and if Modi does not make good on his commitments to achieve universal health coverage in the next few years, a day of reckoning will not be far away.

References

1 Govindarajan V. and Ramamurti R., 'Delivering world-class care affordably,' *Harvard Business Review* (2013).

2 Ibid.

3 World Bank, Government-sponsored health insurance in India: Are you covered? (World Bank, 2012).

4 Ministry of Health and Family Welfare, National Health Policy 2015 – Draft (MOHFW India, 2014), p. 8.

5 Ibid.

6 Unicef statistics, % of children under five underweight (Unicef, 2014).

7 World Bank statistics, Mortality rate under 5 (per 1,000 live births) (World Bank, 2013).

8 World Bank statistics, Improved sanitation facilities (% of population with access) (World Bank, 2012).

9 World Bank statistics, Health expenditure per capita (World Bank, 2012).

10 Ministry of Health and Family Welfare, National Health Policy 2015 – Draft (MOHFW India, 2014).

11 World Bank statistics, Rural population (% of total population) (World Bank, 2013).

12 India National Census statistics, Infant mortality rate by state (Ministry of Home Affairs, 2012).

13 Ministry of Health and Family Welfare, National Health Policy 2015 – Draft (MOHFW India, 2014).

14 PWC, Enabling access to long-term finance for healthcare in India (PWC, 2013), p. 7.

15 Kalra A., India's universal healthcare rollout to cost $26bn (Reuters, 30 October 2014).

16 Kalra A., Deserted New Delhi hospitals sour India's healthcare dream (Reuters, 12 February 2015).

17 PWC, Enabling access to long-term finance for healthcare in India (PWC, 2013).

Middle East and Africa

11 Qatar
Build and they will come

Like many parts of the Middle East, Qatar's natural resource wealth in hydrocarbons has propelled the country on to the global stage and raised the ambitions of its citizens and residents alike. Winning the competition to host the 2022 FIFA World Cup has brought a palpable sense of excitement to this small country with big designs. In political, economic and social affairs, Qatar is becoming increasingly prominent across the Gulf region.

With a population of 2.3 million, three-quarters of which is male, Qatar covers just 11,600 square kilometres – a little over half the size of Wales. More than 94 per cent of the workforce is foreign,[1] leaving about 250,000 Qatari citizens who now have one of the highest average incomes per capita in the world, standing at US$93,397 in 2014.[2] As one of the world's largest suppliers of liquefied natural gas, Qatar intends to continue investing aggressively across sectors. The National Development Strategy 2011–16 is a plan to invest US$200 billion from its sizeable budget surpluses in around 200 large government projects aimed at diversifying the economy away from its current reliance on hydrocarbon revenues. It is becoming a primary destination for global companies who want to be a part of this expansion.

This vision is reflected in the National Health Strategy for 2011–16.[3] It has the potential to bring about substantial change to the system which currently spends around 2.2 per cent of its GDP on health.[4] Its ambition is to provide nothing less than 'a comprehensive world-class health care system whose services are accessible to the whole population'.

The National Health Strategy is intended to improve health services through seven key objectives: ensuring high-quality care is accessible to everyone; integrating services; encouraging preventative measures; building a more skilled workforce; creating effective regulation; managing costs; and expanding the amount of world-class medical research.

Qatar aims to be the premier centre for medical research in the Gulf and is prepared to pay top prices for leading individuals and teams – all backed up by a new Qatar Medical Research Council and the globally recognised Qatar Foundation, which has recently sponsored the Qatar Science and Technology

Park, a US$300 million free trade zone for innovative technology companies. Additional healthcare-focused research will be accommodated in the Sidra Medical and Research Center to 'translate the results from the centre's basic research into something that can be used in the interests of the patients'.

The Sidra Center, now due to open during 2017/18, exemplifies the ambition of Qatar's health service. Its construction is being backed by a US$7.1 billion endowment from the Qatar Foundation and will offer healthcare for women and children locally and across the Gulf. Equipment will include 'smart beds' that keep patients moving to prevent pressure sores, automated vehicles to transport goods around the hospital and palm-scanning authentication technology to store patient records. It will employ more than 5,000 people including 2,000 nurses and 600 doctors. Many of the staff will be drawn from the US and Canada, with around one in seven expected to come from the UK.[5]

The expansion of research complements the rapid investment in hospital facilities. The health sector is overseen by the Supreme Council for Health and the hospital sector is dominated by the Hamad Medical Corporation (HMC), founded in 1979. The HMC runs three general and five specialist hospitals as well as the national ambulance service and a home healthcare service, but a major building and refurbishment programme is underway, including the 216,000 square metre Hamad Medical City. The expansion in capacity shows Qatar's goal of becoming a regional destination for health services, although to some extent it is also playing catch-up – its current bed ratio is low at 1.2 per 1,000 compared with an OECD average of 4.8.[6]

While some services already match the best in the world, there is poor coordination between Qatar's hospitals and clinics. This leads to uneven care quality and makes it difficult to share patient information, although the main providers are rolling out a shared clinical information system which will, in time, lead to a single patient record. In response to the lack of any objective systems for comparing providers' performance, the Supreme Council for Health is now establishing a standard set of measures against which all providers will have to report.

Finding the Staff

The education, training and recruitment of vast numbers of healthcare workers is underway but poses a significant challenge to the strategic vision. A new Medical School at Qatar University will open in 2015 while Weill Cornell Medical College, part of Cornell University in the US, already trains doctors locally. Canada's University of Calgary is providing education and training facilities for nurses. Yet, only around 10 per cent of the nation's existing healthcare workforce is Qatari, a proportion that the government would like to expand. While some progress has been made for higher-paid roles, such as doctors, with such a high average per capita income it is not clear what inducements the government can offer Qataris to select nursing or allied health professions over other better-paid and less onerous training schemes.

In the meantime, a huge global search and selection process has been launched with professional connections being made across Europe, Asia and North America. In a world which is short of well-trained, qualified health clinicians and technicians, the sheer scale of ambition in Qatar will be attractive to many. But the strategy is, of course, high risk. The philosophy of 'build and they will come' is not without its limitations. They may fail to attract the number and quality they want and a large majority of those recruited can be expected to view Qatar as a temporary lucrative placement which will make it hard to build and retain skills.

Hospital Dominance

There are other risks too. While the National Health Strategy has seven important goals set across 35 key programmes, it appears that the desire to promote national pride and ambition is concentrating energy and resources on building hospitals. Primary, community and ambulatory care is relatively weak and the health sector is dominated by a single hospital provider. I was told that over half a million visits to the emergency room take place every year, making the HMC emergency facilities among the busiest in the world. While the country's various building programmes and traffic give rise to a sizeable number of accidents, many visits to the emergency room concern non-communicable diseases and long-term conditions which could easily be cared for outside of hospital. The strategic plan is clear that this needs to happen but, like many systems which have been designed in the twentieth century, the pull of the secondary and tertiary care system could prove a distraction.

The National Health Strategy is developing a regulatory system covering professionals, safety, healthcare quality, products and pharmaceuticals. With a nod to cumbersome attempts elsewhere in the world, the strategy notes that it must 'establish a clear and comprehensive regulatory framework that monitors the healthcare system, ensuring safety and quality, yet not impeding positive progress'.[7]

Goal Six of the National Health Strategy has the rather euphemistic title 'Effective and affordable services, partnership in the bearing of costs'. Simply put, the government wants employers to take a greater role in the financing of healthcare so that the system becomes self-sustaining.

Although Qatar has vast national wealth and could easily afford to fund a fully public service, it wants to create a contestable system which promotes competition between hospitals and the public and private sectors. In a radical move which has stimulated much discussion, the Supreme Council for Health is creating a national insurance programme.

The New Insurance Scheme

The first phase of the insurance scheme, known as Seha, began in July 2013 with coverage for Qatari national women. The full scheme should be in place sometime after 2016. It will eventually provide citizens and residents with 'comprehensive health insurance coverage for all their basic healthcare needs', according to the National Health Insurance Company, the government-owned body that operates Seha.

The Supreme Council of Health will set the prices, which should curb the excessive rates charged by some private services. Patients will have the right to visit any public or private hospital and services beyond the basic package will be available through additional private insurance. Cover for overseas staff is intended to be provided by their employers.

Private healthcare insurance reinforces the message of competition between providers. Its introduction has been viewed with consternation in some quarters but it is clear there is a significant appetite for further investment from the private sector. Government authorities understand the importance of greater private sector participation and the National Development Strategy seeks to increase private hospital beds in the country from 20 per cent to 25 per cent in the next few years.[8] In 2010, 91 new private ambulatory clinics opened, which may well be a sign of the future. New data sources, performance management techniques and tariffs will need to be introduced to make the market work effectively.

Demand may be increased further by the growing problem of obesity and diabetes. More than 70 per cent of Qataris are overweight and more than 40 per cent are obese, pushing Qatar towards the top of the global obesity league.[9] Roughly half of Qataris report low levels of physical activity.[10] This is partly attributable to the sedentary lifestyle which goes with the exceptionally high income, while the extreme desert heat presents a formidable barrier to outdoor exercise for much of the year. The population is young, so the full effects of unhealthy behaviours will not be apparent for some time; however, chronic diseases tend to begin earlier among Middle Eastern peoples, so they may not be that far down the line.

The influx of skilled and unskilled workers to Qatar and the expansion of healthcare facilities is so rapid that reliable estimates of the growth in healthcare demand in the next few years are impossible to come by but an annual figure between 10 per cent and 15 per cent seems likely. With expat workers constituting such a large part of the Qatari population, the rollout of the health programme to foreign workers from 2016 onwards could well prove its most difficult test.

This is a critical issue for the foreign workers known as SMLs – single male labourers – who account for around 45 per cent of Qatar's workforce. Typically aged 20–45 and working in physically demanding and often high-risk jobs in an extreme climate, their medical needs need to be addressed. Among the measures to address this is the construction of three hospitals,[11] but with fewer than 400 beds between them this is nowhere near the scale of what needs to be done.

Conclusion

The sheer scale of ambition for Qatar and its health service is impressive by any global standards. Its comprehensive National Health Strategy discusses all the right things but, as ever, actions speak louder than words. If the health system is to be sustainable in the long term, when economic conditions may be more difficult for the country, more attention will need to be given to expanding and developing local domestic clinical talent and a vibrant primary care sector. Making all this happen at the extraordinary speed demanded by the Qatari government will require the use of the most advanced e-health systems and the best global management skills.

Let us hope that the global lessons of twentieth-century healthcare are digested so that Qatar creates a system which is much more than the magnificence of its buildings.

References

1 Qatar Statistics Authority (2012).

2 World Bank, GDP per capita (current US$) (World Bank, 2014).

3 Supreme Council of Health, National Health Strategy 2011–16: Caring for the future: 2014 Update (State of Qatar, 2014).

4 World Bank statistics, Total health expenditure (% GDP) (World Bank, 2013).

5 Roberts E., Qatar offers thousands of expat jobs at pioneering medical centre (*The Telegraph*, 21 May 2014).

6 World Bank statistics, Hospital beds (per 1,000 people) (World Bank, 2012).

7 Supreme Council of Health, National Health Strategy 2011–16: Caring for the future: 2014 Update (State of Qatar, 2014).

8 Supreme Council of Health, National Health Strategy 2011–16: Caring for the future: 2014 Update (State of Qatar, 2014).

9 Supreme Council of Health, Qatar Health Report 2012 (State of Qatar, 2012).

10 Supreme Council of Health, Qatar Health Report 2012 (State of Qatar, 2012).

11 Supreme Council of Health (1 April 2014).

12 Israel
The best kept secret in global health?

By any international standards, Israel has a good health system. Among all the countries I have worked in, Israel has one of the most progressive primary care services, ably facilitated by their health maintenance organisations (HMOs).

With a population of just over eight million, Israel has long produced good comparative healthcare outcomes on a range of indicators – low infant mortality, high life expectancy, effective chronic disease management and excellent primary care. These results are consistent with the country's longstanding commitment to community and family practice medicine, all provided through a strong public health orientation. Israel boasts one of the highest life expectancy levels in the OECD, with an average of 82.1 years.[1] Its GDP spend on healthcare is a modest 7.2 per cent[2] compared with the OECD average of 9.2 per cent. The Israeli health system can be seen as a high-performing blend of state-inspired universal healthcare with liberal choice.

Worker Roots

Understanding the Israeli health system requires an appreciation of the history of the Zionist movement and the creation of the state. The labour and other Zionist pioneer movements were instrumental in setting the tone for universal healthcare and the Bismarckian social insurance that exists today. In 1911, the Labor Federation of Agricultural Workers founded Clalit as a mutual aid healthcare society. The idea to establish it followed an accident in an orchard in which labourer Baruch Priver lost an arm. It was affiliated to the Histadrut labour movement and mirrored some of the Friendly Societies which had been created across Europe. After 1948 the Clalit and Maccabi HMOs became important parts of the healthcare system of the new state of Israel. A series of healthcare reforms in the following decades led to the HMOs building up substantial deficits. To prevent them sliding into bankruptcy the National Health Insurance Law was passed in 1995, ensuring universal healthcare for both citizens and permanent residents.

The 1995 Act made membership of one of the four existing HMOs – Clalit, Maccabi, Leumit and Meuhedet – compulsory, although citizens can choose which one to join, and the law determined a uniform benefits package available to all, irrespective of age or health status. This insurance-based system is financed with earmarked taxes and contributions paid out of salaries at a progressive rate, supplemented by state funding. Premiums are collected by the National Insurance Institute and are transferred to the four non-government, not-for-profit HMOs based on a capitation formula, who then purchase and provide services. Citizens can top up their mandatory insurance by paying a premium to access additional services from the HMO or through private insurance. The supplementary insurance through the HMOs, called Shaban, is government-approved and bought through a fixed membership fee established according to age rather than health risk.

This system has resulted in government spending on healthcare amounting to just 60 per cent of the total,[3] some way below the OECD average of 72 per cent. Consequently, pressures have been building in the system for some time as the relatively low spending creates inequality in access to healthcare among the population.

All the HMOs have developed primary care at scale, with general practitioners and specialist physicians delivering care from the same settings. The largest HMO, Clalit, is *the* major health organisation in Israel and one of the most progressive public health organisations in the world. It provides care to over half the population and acts as both an insurer and provider. Running 1,400 primary care clinics and eight hospitals providing roughly a third of the country's beds, alongside a countrywide network of pharmacies, dental clinics, laboratories, diagnostic imaging and specialist centres, it can claim to be a fairly self-contained health system which provides excellent care at low cost. If Clalit was based in the US, the entire world would have heard of its success and been studying its formula.

Sophisticated Technology

Part of the success of Clalit and Maccabi rests on their early adoption of technology, for both patient choice and care; during my most recent visit the Clalit medical director justifiably boasted that nearly 60 per cent of all paediatric consultations were now taking place over smartphones. He was clear that the success of the HMO was based on the cooperation between family doctor and hospital specialist to provide a 'medical-social perspective for the care of the individual, the family and the community'.

They invested intensively in online personal medical records which enable the patient and specialist to engage in discussion, treatment and follow-up, and have developed innovative telemedicine programmes which complement Israel's position as a global technology innovator.

The primary care-led HMO system developed in Israel is a great case study for many countries trying to develop a cheaper, less hospital-dominated model of care for the twenty-first century. The trend is to try to shift part of the treatment to the community while strengthening communications between community services and hospitals. However, it would be wrong to suggest that all is well. The double role of the government as both regulator and hospital owner, the strength of the HMOs as purchaser and the scaled-up primary care have combined to put hospitals in a difficult position.

Hospitals – The Weaker Link

This is mirrored in public perceptions of healthcare in Israel. Polls suggest that 90 per cent of Israelis express high levels of satisfaction with both their primary care physicians and their basic health plans but their satisfaction with acute and hospital care is much lower.[4] They express concern about quality, access, the cost of hospital admissions and long waiting times. These concerns have fuelled the uptake of additional health insurance, which has started to challenge the efficiency and effectiveness of the whole system.

Israel has among the lowest proportion of acute-care hospital beds in the OECD. With an average of 3.1 beds per 1,000 people – compared with an OECD average of 4.8[5] – the occupancy rate stands at a staggering 96 per cent compared with an OECD average of 76 per cent.[6] Having run several hospitals in the UK with occupancy rates of over 85 per cent, I sympathise with hospital managers and clinicians who complain that throughput is too quick and, on occasions, unsafe. The average length of stay in Israel is 4.3 days compared with an OECD average of 6.5 days.[7] Lengthy waiting lists indicate this combination of few beds and high occupancy is unsustainable.

The Israeli health system is kept remarkably lean – sometimes to a fault – through funding pressures designed to keep hospital and HMO costs low. As a result, the HMOs run up persistent deficits which have often required cost-cutting and delayed payments to providers. In the end, the state usually picks up the bill so the Treasury is exerting pressure to keep costs down. An inescapable issue is Israel's high defence spending; in Europe, health has been one of the main beneficiaries of the 'peace dividend' following the end of the Cold War.

Striking Doctors

There have been a number of high-profile consequences of financial restraint. Numerous doctor strikes have sought to improve conditions, hours and pay. After a large strike in 2011, a nine-year agreement was implemented to settle matters, although it is far from clear whether it will succeed. A new medical school will increase the supply of much-needed graduates: Israel benefited from the immigration of a large number of former Soviet Union physicians in the 1990s but this cohort is now ageing and most doctors are aged over 55.[8]

Hospitals regularly incur deficits, notably the US$360m debt run up by the huge Hadassah Medical Organization, a non-profit, non-government hospital provider run by the Women's Zionist Organization of America. Problems include rising labour costs after years of pay increases, expanding benefits and growing staff numbers. Many Israeli doctors have two or more public and private jobs, so the public and private sectors are competing for doctors' time while the total working hours are long – a 2003 study put the average figure at 63 hours per week.[9] Financial pressures in the hospital sector are leading to a decline in the quality of infrastructure, including facilities, capacity and technology.

Waiting times for surgery are not transparent and an open culture of quality and safety is still developing. There are few public reports about hospital performance and, while choice exists, it is far from informed. Lengthy waiting lists are a major reason for over three-quarters of the population having taken out secondary health insurance,[10] up from just 46 per cent in 1999.[11]

The Battle Over Reform

In 2013, to address the financial and organisational pressures, health minister Yael German embarked on an almost two-year-long review of the nation's healthcare system. Her Committee to Strengthen the Public Healthcare System in Israel called for more funding for health plans alongside additional investment of around US$330 million, all aimed at shortening waiting times, making private insurance less attractive and being able to pay specialists more to lure them back to public hospitals. Information about private health insurance was to be opened up, with plans unbundled and simplified to reduce the incredible waste created by people holding duplicate and overlapping policies.

The German Committee also proposed ways of strengthening patient choice and improving coordination between the health plans and hospitals. It wanted a new National Hospital Authority to manage public hospitals, leaving the Ministry of Health space to focus on being a regulator. Significantly, it recommended prohibiting the expansion of private services in public hospitals, so that people could not buy better services in a taxpayer-funded facility and to avoid the public health system being dependent on private health spending.

The German recommendations encountered stiff political and professional opposition from the start due to the perception they were too heavily focused on propping up hospitals, and the limits proposed on doctors' ability to do private work. Following the general election of March 2015, Yael German was replaced as health minister by Yakhov Litzman. Litzman, who previously held the post between 2009 and 2013, branded her reform proposals 'a total failure' and committed to abolishing '80 per cent' of them.[12] Litzman's direction of travel is likely to be towards increasing the ability of public hospitals to provide private services – which would raise much needed revenue for the acute sector, but has sparked concerns about the system becoming less equal. Litzman has also suggested he will move to broaden the basic basket of health services available to all to include some aged care services, to be funded by a 0.5 per cent rise in the health tax.

There are significant health inequalities in Israel, especially for Arab Israelis. As well as income disparities, these inequalities are partly caused by the strikingly high levels of smoking among Arab Israeli men, and the high incidence of obesity among Arab Israeli women. Alongside Arab Israelis, the ultra-orthodox Haredi account for a significant share of the country's poverty. Both Arab and ultra-orthodox communities are growing fast, accounting for around a third of the population and half of the children entering primary school.

Among its other health challenges, Israel has the second-highest rate of skin cancers in the world after Australia – a by-product of Jewish immigration from cooler European countries.[13]

Conclusion

Countries around the world could learn from Israel's healthcare system. The legacy of population health and community care is a key contributor to the country's impressive achievements in outcomes and life expectancy. But it risks undermining these successes built over decades unless it reforms its hospital system and makes strategic investments to stem rising dissatisfaction and financial instability.

References

1 World Bank statistics, Life expectancy at birth (World Bank, 2013).

2 World Bank statistics, Total health expenditure (% of GDP) (World Bank, 2013).

3 OECD, OECD Health Statistics 2014: How does Israel compare? (OECD, 2012).

4 OECD, OECD Reviews of healthcare quality: Israel (OECD, 2012).

5 OECD, OECD Health Statistics 2014: How does Israel compare? (OECD, 2014).

6 Economist Intelligence Unit, Industry Report, Healthcare (EIU, September 2014), p. 8.

7 EIU (2014), p. 8.

8 OECD, OECD Health Statistics 2014: How does Israel compare? (OECD, 2012).

9 Nirel N. et al., Physician Specialists in Israel: Modes of Employment and the Implications for Their Work (JDC, Brookdale Institute: Jerusalem, 2003).

10 Hemmings P., 'How to Improve Israel's Health-care System,' OECD, Paper No. 1114 (April 2014).

11 Bowers L., 'Hot Issues in Israel's Healthcare System,' in *Taub Center for Social Policy Studies in Israel, Policy Brief* (March 2014).

12 Sharon J., Litzman: We will roll back measures against Haredi community from last government (*The Jerusalem Post*, 19 March 2015).

13 EIU (2014), p. 13.

13 South Africa
No more false dawns

Healthcare in Africa is changing. While the continent still shoulders the greatest burden of communicable diseases and struggles to provide clean water and sanitation, its economic growth – which averaged around 6 per cent over the last decade – is lifting millions out of poverty and creating an urban middle class and a more assertive population among the poor, who are demanding more from their governments on healthcare. Calls for universal health cover grow ever louder and are being keenly pursued by Nigeria, Tunisia, Ethiopia, Ghana, Rwanda and South Africa among others.

The 'double burden' of disease facing Africa is increasingly recognised by governments, with WHO estimating that by 2030 chronic diseases will overtake communicable ones as the most common cause of death.[1] But there remains a huge unfinished agenda across the continent. Progress towards the Millennium Development Goals has been far slower than hoped and, so far, the gap between Africa and the rest of the world grows only wider: maternal mortality in Africa is currently declining at 1.7 per cent a year, against 2.3 per cent worldwide and 5 per cent in South East Asia.[2]

Nevertheless, there is an undeniable sense of optimism across many parts of the continent and experimentation with new care models is taking place to reach as many people as possible with the very limited resources available. For example, over the past decade Ethiopia has rapidly expanded access to primary care to around 85 per cent of the population, contributing to a stunning 52 per cent reduction in infant mortality. Tunisia has developed a near-universal coverage system based on employee contributions and government subsidies and Rwanda's achievements in going from the ruins of genocide to socially inclusive universal health coverage are equally remarkable.

South Africa's Journey to Universal Healthcare

South Africa is an 'exception to the rule' in so many ways to the rest of the continent. However, much of this spirit of optimism can be found there too – albeit with a number of false dawns along the way. The end of apartheid in 1994 threw a spotlight on the huge health inequalities in the country and the African National Congress government has made several attempts since to improve cover for the 84 per cent of the population reliant on the public healthcare system. The most promising of these efforts is currently underway: a 14-year strategy for a comprehensive National Health Insurance (NHI) system to cover 48 million people. The NHI is part of a wider 10-point plan to improve public hospitals, health infrastructure, the quality and quantity of health workers, and reduce HIV and maternal deaths. Pilots have begun and progress is being made but the prospect of universal health coverage has provoked fierce debate as to who will pay – just 5 million of South Africa's 53 million citizens pay income tax.[3]

South Africa currently spends a respectable 8.9 per cent of its GDP on healthcare;[4] however, half of this goes towards just 16 per cent of the population that can afford private insurance.[5] There is a tenfold difference in the spending on health for the privately insured (US$1,500 per capita per annum) compared with those receiving care in the public sector (US$150 per capita per annum).[6] This creates huge disparities in care and explains why South Africa's respectable average spending on health produces such poor outcomes relative to other countries: life expectancy is just 57 years compared with 74, 71, 66 and 75 in the other BRICS countries – Brazil, Russia, India and China respectively.[7]

Implementing the NHI will require a major scale-up in public funding for healthcare. In 2012–13 this stood at R121 billion (US$40 billion) but at full implementation the scheme has been projected to cost R336 billion per year (US$111 billion) by 2025–6.[8]

People and Buildings

Of course, health financing is just one of a number of factors that have held back South Africa and which it must overcome to achieve healthcare for all. Recruiting and retaining clinical staff is an enduring problem, with vacancy rates for doctor and nursing posts reported to be 56 per cent and 46 per cent respectively.[9] Shortages are particularly serious in rural areas; half the population lives there, but only 3 per cent of doctors graduating every year take jobs in the countryside.[10] The quality of health workers is also a concern, with the private sector attracting 70 per cent of South Africa's newly qualified doctors through better pay and conditions[11] despite all medical training being done in the public sector.

To counter this, salaries for public health workers and training capacity have been expanded. Medical student numbers increased by 34 per cent between 2000 and 2012, partly driven by controversial 'affirmative action' policies that increased entry of black and female students with lower academic scores.[12] The government has been negotiating overseas to discourage other countries from 'poaching' its health workers. A deal with the UK has led to a significant reduction in South African nurses working there but other countries, aware of their own staff shortages, have often been less amenable. South Africa, in turn, has turned to overseas labour markets to plug its gap: around 10 per cent of doctors qualified overseas, especially in other African countries (with their own workforce shortages), Cuba and Iran. The country is also innovating in the face of doctor shortages, bringing new cadres of 'paraprofessionals' such as clinical health associates, community health workers and patients and communities themselves into the workforce.

The government has stated that the care in public hospitals needs to improve, from both a capacity and quality perspective. Many are poorly equipped and what equipment they have is poorly maintained. Public–private partnerships are developing, such as funding for private sector care of public patients.

Some 200 clinics are being built and the government has promised to refurbish and re-equip hundreds more in the 11 pilot districts of the NHI. New hospitals are also planned. There are currently more than 400 public hospitals and over 200 private ones, with mining companies running their own hospitals.

Fragmentation at Every Level

The first five years of the NHI will focus on developing the necessary administrative and management infrastructure for a functioning health system and there is certainly much to do. There is fragmentation at almost every level of the public system: the National Department of Health carries overall responsibility for healthcare; provincial health departments manage larger hospitals directly (except for estates which are maintained by their public works departments); and smaller hospitals and primary care are managed in their districts. There are also municipal health services – including public health responsibilities, such as clean water – run by the local authorities, which are separate from the districts. Local authorities also run some primary care clinics but this is being phased out. All this results in poor coördination between primary and secondary services, which encourages patients to bypass primary care and head straight to hospital.

Controversially, the National Department of Health has taken direct management of the country's 10 major academic hospitals from the provincial governments, partly justified through accusations about diversion of training funds to services.

In 2014 the government launched the Office for Health Standards and Compliance to monitor and improve quality standards across public and private sectors and encourage greater innovation in models of care. One of the issues it will address is the quality of management skills, a major challenge which blights the health system and will hold back the NHI if not addressed quickly. Indeed, some have argued that this is the real central problem of South Africa's public health system – not just the lack of resources but its low productivity and waste through inefficient management.[13]

The 'Quadruple' Burden of Disease

While South Africa's progress on health over recent decades compares poorly with emerging economies in Asia and South America, it has had to deal with one health problem of a massive scale. Around 200,000 people still die every year from AIDS in South Africa,[14] which has one of the highest infection rates in the world – 19 per cent of the adult population.[15] The country's early response to the epidemic was a case study in weak, inept policy-making: denial of the virus's existence, waves of programmes never implemented, and rejected offers of grants and donated drugs.

Thankfully, the situation has improved markedly. South Africa now has the largest antiretroviral programme in the world, with 2.2 million people currently accessing treatment costing over US$1 billion per year.[16] A comprehensive national strategy is in place investing in condom distribution, mass testing and public education. Infection rates have finally started falling and major progress has been made in cutting mother-to-child transmission of the disease, which has helped infant mortality rates fall from 54 per 1,000 live births to 33 per 1,000 over the last decade.[17] Still, a huge task remains: 370,000 more South Africans were infected with HIV in 2012,[18] drug-resistant tuberculosis is rapidly on the rise among people with AIDS, and there is early evidence suggesting that the transition of HIV from death sentence to long-term condition is encouraging some people to slip back into risky behaviours, such as unprotected sex.[19]

The catastrophe of HIV/AIDS has forced innovation in the delivery systems of South African healthcare, which the rollout of NHI may capitalise on. For example, the use of nurses to manage and support the antiretroviral programme was a major success. One notable development has been the popularity of mobile testing, such as the Tutu Tester Mobile Clinics launched by the Desmond Tutu HIV Foundation. These combine testing for a range of common communicable and non-communicable diseases using vans that can reach South Africa's remote and underserved areas. Such approaches not only address multiple health problems at once, they also get around the stigma that still exists around going for HIV testing. Another remarkable innovation was the extent to which patients and communities themselves were mobilised, playing a vital role in the scale-up of drug distribution, treatment adherence and public education.

The scale of the communicable disease challenge in South Africa is such that it is often easy to forget the extent of other epidemiological problems facing the country. Lifestyle-related conditions are rising rapidly: around 10 per cent of men and 28 per cent of women were classified as morbidly obese in 2012,[20] and South Africa has an infamously high rate of deaths through injury, including one of the highest homicide rates in the world. The scale of these challenges are such that South Africa has been described as having a 'quadruple' burden of disease: communicable, non-communicable, violence, and maternal and child health.[21]

There is only so much a health system will ever be able to do to overcome these problems. Even if world-class care were available to all, 45 per cent of the population still live on around US$2 per day[22] and the dire problems of poverty and ill health will continue until social and economic development spread.

Private Sector Care

For those that can afford it, however, healthcare in South Africa can be very good. The private healthcare market offers good-quality care to the 16 per cent of the population with access to it. But cover is becoming ever more expensive, with above-inflation rate rises for the past decade. The main drivers for this appear to be the fee-for-service system which many providers are paid on, increasing service use by members and – controversially – claims that the sector is becoming uncompetitive. Three providers dominate, holding around 80 per cent of the private hospital market between them.[23] In 2014 South Africa's Competition Commission began a wide-ranging market inquiry into the sector to investigate its competitiveness and how it could be made more accessible and affordable.

Conclusion

Health systems reflect the societies in which they develop and South Africa is a perfect example. Despite great progress, it remains a deeply divided society with arguably the highest income disparity in the world.[24] This polarity is reflected in healthcare, with a large under-resourced and over-stretched public system alongside a comfortable private hospital sector. With the NHI strategy underway and the competition inquiry launched, both of these poles are likely to face fundamental change in the coming years. There have been false dawns before but momentum is behind the current push for universal coverage. The government will have to deliver this time after its very public promises. What remains to be seen is whether the capacity exists to implement these grand plans and whether they can be combined with the other foundations of a successful society – education, employment and a safe environment.

References

1 World Health Organization African Region, Ministerial consultation on non-communicable diseases (WHO AR, 2011).

2 KPMG Africa, The state of healthcare in Africa (KPMG Africa, 2014).

3 KPMG South Africa, Too few tax payers: What are the implications? (KPMG South Africa, 2013).

4 World Bank statistics, Total health expenditure (% of GDP) (World Bank, 2013).

5 Presidency of the Republic of South Africa, Twenty-year review: 1994–2014 (Republic of South Africa, 2014).

6 Benatar S., 'The challenges of health disparities in South Africa' in *South African Medical Journal*, 103, 3 (2013).

7 World Bank statistics, Life expectancy at birth (World Bank, 2013).

8 Economist Intelligence Unit, Healthcare industry report: South Africa (EIU, 2014).

9 Rondganger L., SA needs 14,531 doctors and 44,780 nurses (*Daily News*, 22 January 2013).

10 Robinson M., SA needs rural doctors (*Mail & Guardian*, 8 April 2014).

11 World Health Organization, 'Bridging the gap in South Africa' in *Bulletin of the World Health Organization*, 88, 11 (WHO, 2010) pp. 797–876.

12 Mayosi B.M. & Benatar S.R., 'Health and health care in South Africa – 20 years after Mandela' in *New England Journal of Medicine*, 371, 14 (2014).

13 Ruff B. et al., 'Reflections on health-care reforms in South Africa' in *Journal of Public Health Policy*, 32 S184–92 (2001).

14 UNAIDS statistics, Deaths due to AIDS (UNAIDS, 2013).

15 World Bank statistics, Prevalence of HIV (population aged 15–49) (World Bank, 2013).

16 Republic of South Africa Department of Health statistics (2013).

17 World Bank statistics, Infant mortality rate (per 1,000 live births) (World Bank, 2013).

18 UNAIDS, New HIV report finds a big drop in new HIV infections in South Africa (UNAIDS, 2014).

19 AVERT, HIV & AIDS in South Africa (AVERT, 2014).

20 Economist Intelligence Unit, Industry Report: Healthcare: South Africa (EIU, 2014).

21 Mayosi B.M. et al., 'The burden of non-communicable disease in South Africa' in *The Lancet*, 374, 9693 (2009) pp. 934–47.

22 Mayosi B.M. and Benatar S.R., 'Health and health care in South Africa – 20 years after Mandela' in *New England Journal of Medicine*, 371, 14 (2014).

23 Holmes T., Hospitals: They're making a killing (*Mail & Guardian*, 14 June 2014).

24 World Bank Statistics, GINI Index (World Bank, 2012).

Europe

14 Russia
A distressed and distressing system

Visiting Russia, I am always struck by the depth of its culture and the enormity of the sacrifices it has made to help win the peace and freedom that Western Europeans like myself now enjoy. I am therefore immensely sad to conclude – like many Russians I have met – that the healthcare system serving this great country has a bleak future.

I must stress that my experiences of Russian healthcare have been confined to Moscow and that, as a federation of 85 states covering the largest area of any nation on earth, it is impossible to generalise too deeply about so large a system from such a narrow lens.

Nevertheless, on recent visits I have become deeply concerned about the state of the Russian healthcare system. This impression is partly a result of Russia's economic situation, which continues to go from bad to worse. At the time of writing, the economy was forecasted to shrink by 5 per cent in 2015. The rouble has lost half its value against the dollar over the last 12 months. Inflation and base rates are around 15 per cent and the ratings agency Standard & Poor's recently downgraded Russia's credit rating to 'junk' status.

In large part, this depressing state of affairs has been driven by the global decline in oil and energy prices, but sanctions in response to Russia's involvement in Ukraine and Crimea are also a major factor – responsible for around 30 per cent of the total fall in government revenue, according to the Minister of Finance.[1] The scale of this impending economic crisis and the country's increasingly isolated geopolitical stance seem to be the dominant forces now shaping Russian health policy, prompting cuts and hasty reforms.

Russia spends a respectable 6.5 per cent of its GDP on healthcare.[2] However, this is channelled through a chaotic system of hierarchically controlled state provision and high levels of out-of-pocket expenditure, with 'unofficial' payments by patients making up a third of all health spending, according to the Economist Intelligence Unit.[3]

On paper, Russia has a mostly free universal healthcare system covering a fairly broad package of services funded by a mix of state, employer and patient contributions. In reality, the constitutional right to healthcare is blocked by opaque and bureaucratic systems of planning and regulation, reimbursement rates for providers that don't cover their costs, a scarcity of resources, and high levels of informal payments to access care in anything approaching a timely manner.

Responsibilities for managing the public system are a 'mosaic' of federal and state-level agencies – the hangover of successive policies decentralising and recentralising functions over the last 25 years. Alongside this, parallel systems of private provision have grown up to provide care for those who can afford it. Overall, around 48 per cent of healthcare spending in Russia comes from government sources, significantly below the OECD average of 72 per cent.[4]

The Soviet Health Race

Russia inherited a healthcare legacy similar to the rest of the former Soviet Union. The Semashko system – based on tiered services hinged on the district physician – led to significant advances in population health during the early and middle twentieth century and was once a commendable attempt at universal coverage. But from the 1970s progress slowed as the government came to see the answer to every health problem as 'more' – more specialists, more facilities, more equipment, more agencies. If the Cold War had been an arms race for healthcare capacity, the Soviet Union would have taken gold medal – by 1985 Russia had around four times the doctors and hospital beds per capita as the US.[5]

Since 1990 some former Soviet states, such as Estonia, have managed to move away from the poorly planned and underutilised system that Semashko became. Unfortunately Russia is not one of these. Attempts to reform the healthcare system have been infrequent and lacklustre, and although bed and doctor numbers have gradually declined, by and large the same overcapacity has been maintained on meagre funding for the last 25 years. During the 1990s and 2000s, Russia's healthcare infrastructure has been in steady decline with increasingly dilapidated facilities, poorly trained doctors and longer waiting times. Around 45 per cent of hospitals are classified as requiring 'major refurbishment', a third lack hot water and 7 per cent don't have a telephone.[6]

This has destroyed trust in the healthcare system in general and doctors in particular. Anton Chekhov's *Ivanov* contains the line, 'doctors – they're just like lawyers, only with doctors when they've finished robbing you, you die'. Despite being written in 1887, this sentiment is one I have heard repeatedly from modern Russians. In a particularly grim recent trend, a spate of suicides among retired military generals has been reported. Unable to access treatment or pain relief for cancers, they take the only course of action available to escape from 'excruciating pain'.[7]

Catastrophic Outcomes

Today, despite spending just US$957 per person on healthcare,[8] Russia still has almost twice the number of beds per thousand as the OECD average (9.3 against 4.8) and around two-thirds more doctors per thousand (4.9 against 3.2).[9] This would be fine if all this capacity was producing better health, but far too much resource is focused on hospitalisation and specialist care and too many doctors are poorly equipped in terms of skills and materials. As a result, the state of the population's health is a catastrophe considering Russia's stage of development. Average life expectancy is 71 years, almost 10 years below the OECD average, putting Russia on a par with Bangladesh and North Korea.[10]

The disparity between male and female life expectancy in Russia is the highest in the world at 65 and 76 years respectively.[11] This 11-year gap is largely due to widespread abuse of alcohol (including 'moonshine'), violence and road accidents. Russia also has a disproportionate problem with HIV/AIDS and related conditions as a result of high levels of intravenous drug use and a lamentably slow acknowledgement of the epidemic by government. Around 59 per cent of men in Russia smoke, the fourth-highest rate in the world.[12]

Russia has set a goal to increase average life expectancy to 75 by 2020. This is a tall mountain to climb and progress towards it so far has been slow. But, as the above figures show, almost the entire target could be met by improving the public health of men. It was a welcome step, then, when in 2014 Russia passed an anti-smoking law in line with global best practice on what works to cut smoking levels.

Wider developments in Russian health policy have been primarily based on political and economic imperatives rather than the health of the population. On his re-election in April 2012, President Putin signed the 'May Decrees', which included a doubling of the wages of healthcare staff by 2018 and gradual privatisation of state health services. A mixed system has been in operation since 1996 anyway, when government health facilities were legally allowed to offer private services, and for-profit providers have been providing state-insured services on a small scale since 2011. But the doubling of health worker wages makes little sense given the problems afflicting Russia's healthcare system. Some commentators have interpreted this as more about strengthening Putin's popular support than improving health, citing one reason for his soaring approval ratings as the consistent increases in benefits to public sector employees throughout his presidency.[13]

Perhaps fortunately, the extent to which the 2012 decrees have been implemented has been limited, a result of healthcare's devolved status and the economic crisis. Moscow has been the first region to make serious changes and in November 2014 the cost of higher wages was hammered home as the closure of 15 hospitals and 13 other health facilities was announced, along with 7,000 redundancies. This led to street protests by health professionals and some local unrest. The policy was paused in response and a review process by a number of oversight bodies has criticised the policy's blunt approach of seeking efficiencies through blanket staff reductions, highlighting the poorer access that has already resulted.

Private Sector Boom

At the same time, the private sector for healthcare in Moscow has been booming. Chains of private clinics have sprung up almost overnight, facilitated by the ease of recruiting recently redundant doctors at competitive salaries and public – private partnerships enabling them to open and operate premises quickly. One rapidly expanding chain – Doktor Ryadom (Doctor Next Door) – uses a mixed model of funding, whereby around half of patients are treated barely at cost under mandatory health insurance and the rest privately. A third option was also launched recently whereby public patients can opt for a policy that offers more free-of-charge services than the normal state guarantee, on the condition that they always receive these at a particular clinic. Although mandatory health insurance reimbursement rates are low, a very few hyper-efficient for-profit clinic providers manage to operate by only seeing state-funded patients.

The quality of some of these private providers appears to be good and they are adding a much-needed surge of innovation to a city whose health system has otherwise been in long-term decline. The services offered are adding capacity where they are most needed, notably primary care, and may go some way to overcoming Russians' deeply engrained suspicion of primary care as second-class medicine. However, Russia remains a difficult place to do business, with banks unwilling to lend and a pervasive sense among companies that, when working with government, 'you never really know the rules of the game'. A number of foreign providers have left the market in the last year.

These factors will limit the growth of these public–private initiatives and it remains to be seen how sustainable they are and what proportion of the population are actually able to access them. Only 5 per cent of Russians have voluntary health insurance, and these are largely confined to the major cities.[14]

Conclusion

Until the economy recovers, a serious appetite for reform and innovation develops, and the cancerous effect of corruption and low public trust are overcome, I see little scope for improvement in Russian healthcare. Partnerships with the private sector provide one ray of hope but it is still without doubt one of the least optimistic systems I have worked in. Regrettably, I do not expect the next few years to bring better news but I hope they will.

References

[1] Spence P., Russia faces recession as oil crash and sanctions cost economy £90bn (*The Telegraph*, 24 November 2014).

[2] World Bank statistics, Total health expenditure (% of GDP) (World Bank, 2013).

[3] Economist Intelligence Unit, Industry report, Healthcare: Russia (EIU, 2014).

[4] World Bank statistics, Public health expenditure (% of total health expenditure) (World Bank, 2012).

[5] Figures from Sharp M.E., *The former Soviet Union in transition* (US Congress Joint Economic Committee: Washington, DC, 1993) and Centres for Disease Control, Healthcare in America: Trends in Utilisation (CDC, 2004).

[6] Popovich L. et al., Russian Federation: Health System Review, Health Systems in Transition 13:7 (European Health Observatory, 2011), p. 96.

[7] Sharkov C., Fourth Russian general commits suicide in less than a year (*Newsweek*, 6 January 2015).

[8] World Bank statistics, Health expenditure per capita (World Bank, 2013).

[9] OECD, Health Statistics 2014: How does the Russian Federation compare (OECD, 2014).

[10] World Bank statistics, Life expectancy at birth (World Bank, 2013).

[11] World Bank statistics, Life expectancy at birth (female and male) (World Bank, 2012).

[12] World Bank statistics, Smoking prevalence, males as percentage of adults (World Bank, 2011).

[13] Institute of Modern Russia, Healthcare reform as a catalyst for progress (IOMR, 2014).

[14] Popovich L. et al., Russian Federation: Health System Review, Health Systems in Transition 13:7 (European Health Observatory, 2011), p. 88.

15 The Nordics Decentralised welfare utopia?

While the 25 million people spread across the enormous area of Iceland, Finland, Denmark, Norway and Sweden do not have homogeneous characteristics, they share many cultural attributes which have shaped their respective, and collective, welfare systems. The Scandinavian countries of Sweden, Denmark and Norway were united in the Kalmar Union from 1397 to 1523 and continued to be united in various constellations, punctuated by numerous wars, before all gained independence during the twentieth century. The Scandinavian model of the welfare state has become internationally recognised and widely generalised but there are some centrifugal forces at play which deserve closer scrutiny.

First, the similarities. The Scandinavian model is characterised by the state playing a dominant role in the formulation of welfare policy and a dominant public sector delivering services to citizens who pay high taxes in return for social cohesion and well-being. Nordic health systems are built on the same principles of universalism, expressing a strong desire for equity regardless of class, race or place of residence. Furthermore, Scandinavian countries have been admired for their decentralised welfare model, where local – municipal or county – political bodies are responsible for raising some taxes, providing some health services and running hospitals.

Impressive Outcomes

While the idealised model above is changing, there is little doubt that the fundamental strengths of the Nordic welfare system have produced good health and well-regarded healthcare. Broadly speaking, spending an average of 9.6 per cent of GDP[1] on healthcare, with average life expectancy at just over 81 years,[2] the Nordic countries can claim impressive OECD performance for many health outcomes including cancer, circulatory conditions and heart disease. In many instances, they have excellent quality registers and well-considered care programmes which are joined up effectively between national, regional and municipal authorities. Some of the Nordic countries also have a long tradition of involving users to improve the quality of care through the use of patient experience measures. Their work on prevention and health promotion is sophisticated and ambitious, as demonstrated in 2014 when the Nordic countries signed the Trondheim Declaration, committing them to stronger collaboration to achieve equitable health and well-being in their region and reduce global health inequities.[3] Their health promotion activities are defined not only by great inter-agency collaboration but excellent cooperation across sectors, often delivered through active localism.

It would be easy to conclude that well-funded healthcare, coupled with active health promotion, coherent national policies and high clinical standards, all implemented through great inter-agency and cross-sector local collaboration, is the perfect recipe for success. However, the reality across the Nordic countries is somewhat different, with variations in system governance, trends towards centralisation, growing involvement of the private sector and an increasing element of co-payment to ensure universality.

Erosion of Local Control

Despite the relative affluence of Scandinavia (especially Norway, with one of the highest GDPs per capita in the world thanks to abundant energy supplies), concerns surrounding cost containment and efficiency are gradually reshaping traditional systems and common-held norms in healthcare. Currently, the Scandinavian model of decentralised local governance has taken at least three different directions. Norway has taken responsibility for hospital services from small, local governments to the state while Denmark has merged counties into fewer, larger regions; this strengthens central control but leaves regionally elected politicians in charge. Sweden maintains its 21-county governance system but has injected significant elements of contestability and patient choice.

In Norway, for example, health spending has accelerated way beyond its Nordic neighbours. While it is comparable as a percentage of GDP, per capita spending stands at roughly US$9,715 per annum, the highest in the world. This contrasts sharply with Denmark (US$6,270), Sweden (US$5,680), Finland (US$4,449) and Iceland (US$4,126).[4] Norway's substantial spending per person provides useful supporting data for those who argue that there is little correlation between per capita health spend and outcomes. Life expectancy is similar across the Nordic countries and they all have waiting time and waiting list problems to a certain extent.

In Denmark, a novel financial stability law was passed in 2012 requiring all regions and municipalities to keep within 1.5 per cent of their budgets, which had to be agreed with the national government. This de facto national veto on the ability of municipalities to set their own 'tax and spend' policies has reduced their levels of responsibility significantly. In addition, the recent hospital-building programme across the five regional authorities seeks to centralise specialist work on the grounds of quality and cost and now requires central government approval, including decisions on the location of new facilities and the closure of old ones. The majority of capital funds now come from centrally held budgets and the regions have lost their tax-raising powers.

In Finland, the government is proposing a seismic restructure of its highly decentralised health and care system by merging the 320 municipalities into five regions through its Reform in Local Government Structures strategy. The argument follows similar lines to those above – scale, speed and scope of services offered. Additionally, the associated Health and Social Care Reform Initiative seeks to open up services to private healthcare companies and provide greater choice. It is anticipated that the new regions, based around the five university hospitals in Finland, would integrate services, standardise care better, reduce bureaucracy and reduce costs to close the 'welfare gap'. While this strategy has not yet been enacted in law – and will, no doubt, face municipal and public opposition – it is likely that many parts of the reform package will be phased in from 2016.

Growth of Contestability

Perhaps the most radical departure from the Scandinavian consensus surrounds the involvement of the private sector in Sweden. While the 21 councils still have responsibility for providing health and care services, the national government up until 2014 embarked on a major reform programme to introduce contestability, choice and financial discipline to the healthcare system. Under the so-called 'Stockholm model', county councils commission care from a mixture of public and private providers. In 2007, Stockholm County Council decided to give patients a free choice of primary care provider. This was followed by a central government decision in 2010 that all county councils should allow free choice, giving private companies the right to set up large GP-style services anywhere in the country – and to be paid for them out of taxpayers' money. Since then, firms have established around 200 GP-style healthcare centres, most of which are in the wealthier areas.[5] It is now estimated that 12 per cent of county council healthcare expenditure is on independent organisations.[6] The figure is considerably more for aged and residential care, also commissioned by councils.

Health and the policy of contestability figured prominently in the 2014 Swedish general election in the wake of several care scandals. Prime Minister Stefan Lofven leads a centre-left coalition but has pledged to 'govern from the centre', thus curbing speculation that private sector firms would be banned from making a profit. However, he stated his intention to better regulate how private companies run public healthcare services and made it clear that 'the pursuit of profit cannot be the overriding motivation' for the sector.[7]

Co-payments are figuring more prominently in Scandinavian countries than the casual observer may have thought. While all Nordic countries bar Finland easily exceed 80 per cent for public sector expenditure on healthcare (OECD average 72 per cent, Finland 75 per cent),[8] there is little need for private insurance systems which, consequently, places a much higher burden on out-of-pocket expenses. Co-payments exist across Scandinavia and Finland, while Norway and Sweden have introduced outpatient consultation charges. Hospital charges are also levied in Sweden. In 2014 the Commonwealth Fund found that 4 per cent of Swedes and 6 per cent of Norwegians reported having problems paying for healthcare.[9] While these figures are low (only the UK performs better at 1 per cent) they nonetheless demonstrate that even Scandinavia struggles with ensuring access is only dependent on need and not ability to pay.

The highly decentralised structure of Nordic health services and taxes can make cost management difficult, as regional and national authorities can argue about whose problem it is to solve. However, having the same decentralised body funding healthcare and raising taxes arguably creates a closer link between funding and ability to pay than, for example, the NHS in England, where local health systems are pressing national government for more cash.

The strong democratic traditions in the Nordic countries are reflected in the way health services are managed. This 'democratic management' approach is characterised by legitimising decisions through the involvement of a wide range of interest groups including patient representatives, trade unions, local politicians and primary care representatives. It is not uncommon for a decentralised approach to work its way into the running of departments and wards, even where there is, in theory, centralised management control. This takes time and decisions are not always made quickly.

The Risks of Fragmentation

Sweden is finding that its ageing population is testing its ability to deliver high-quality care and risks paying a price for its fragmented system. The OECD has found that one of the country's biggest challenges is securing effective coordination of care between hospitals, primary care and local authorities.[10] This is one of the few areas in which Sweden compares poorly in international studies. It sees greater central control as part of the solution, with national quality standards and sharing of outcome data, particularly around GPs and elderly care services.

The OECD states: 'In many ways, Sweden's health and long-term care systems are regarded as exemplars to be emulated across the OECD. Yet an ageing population, increasing expectations of service users and diversification in how, where and when care is delivered are testing these systems' ability to continue delivering high quality care.'[11]

The problem is not so much structure as poor coordination along clinical pathways. Sweden has developed guidelines for a minority of conditions, such as dementia, schizophrenia and substance abuse, but needs to extend its focus to support many more patients, alongside minimum quality standards. This in itself runs counter to Sweden's preference for encouragement rather than direction but there is evidence that the public is increasingly valuing consistency in quality over local diversity. The country has built extensive registers of service quality on which minimum standards can be built.

The OECD highlights the risks of the recent reforms promoting competition and choice causing further fragmentation of services for patients with complex needs.[12] For example, since 2010 every patient has had the right to choose between a public and private provider in primary care. This could dilute the counties' clear local responsibility for population health. Attempts to increase choice by allowing businesses to set up clinics in both primary and specialist care are being undermined by political resistance from the county councils.

But, despite these problems, Sweden's health record is impressive. It has one of the lowest infant mortality rates in the world,[13] one of the highest cancer survival rates,[14] has the lowest smoking rates in the OECD and low obesity.[15] Health inequalities are also low and the quality of long-term care is among the best globally.

Conclusion

While healthcare leaders in other countries will find some reassurance in the fact that even the Nordic countries are finding it difficult to cope with ageing populations, their overall health performance still sets a standard which few are likely to match in the near future. Their healthcare systems are an expression of their values of social cohesion and equity, secured by relatively high taxation. Their biggest challenge is to remain true to their values while reforming their health economies to ensure they can continue to provide outstanding service in the coming decades.

References

1 World Bank statistics, Total health expenditure (% of GDP), (World Bank, 2013).

2 World Bank statistics, Life expectancy at birth, (World Bank, 2013).

3 Trondheim Declaration: Equity in health and wellbeing – a political choice (11th Nordic Health Promotion Conference, 27–29 August 2014).

4 World Bank statistics, Health expenditure per capita (World Bank, 2013).

5 Bidgood E., Healthcare systems: Sweden and localism – an example for the UK? (Civitas, 2013).

[6] Economist Intelligence Unit, Industry Report, Healthcare (EIU, December 2013), p. 7.

[7] Duxbury C, New Swedish Premier names ministers and sets out policy, (*Wall Street Journal*, 3 October 2014).

[8] World Bank, Health expenditure, public (% of total health expenditure) (World Bank, 2012).

[9] Commonwealth Fund, Mirror on the wall: How the performance of the US healthcare system performs internationally – 2014 Update (Commonwealth Fund: New York, 2014).

[10] OECD, OECD Reviews of healthcare quality: Sweden – Raising standards (OECD, 2013).

[11] OECD (2013).

[12] OECD (2013).

[13] OECD, Infant mortality (Deaths per 1,000 live births) (OECD, 2012).

[14] OECD, Breast cancer five-year relative survival (OECD, 2011).

[15] OECD, OECD Health Statistics 2014: How does Sweden compare? (OECD, 2014), p. 3.

16 The Netherlands Competition and social solidarity

In some quarters, the Dutch healthcare system is rated the best in the world. It has topped the Commonwealth Fund performance table[1] and the EuroHealth Consumer Index for patient-centredness,[2] while boasting a pioneering spirit of reform which combines competition with social solidarity.

A relatively small country, with 16 million inhabitants, the Netherlands' health system has been heavily influenced by the Bismarck school of social insurance. It was created in 1941 during the German occupation, when the first Sickness Fund Decree was introduced. Much later, under the banner of social solidarity, the 2006 Health Insurance Act (Zvw) abolished the distinction between mandatory sickness fund insurance and voluntary private insurance which had existed since the Second World War. In doing so, the Zvw fundamentally changed the role of government from directly controlling healthcare volume, prices and productive capacity to 'setting the rules of the game' and regulating the newly formed market.

Managed competition for providers and insurers has become the major driver in the healthcare system and has heralded fundamental changes for patients, providers, insurers and government. In this sense, the Dutch system presents a unique variant – a health system which believes in both social solidarity and competition, and with the public and private sectors working together.

All residents have to take out health insurance, costing roughly €1,100–€1,200 a year. Insurers are obliged to accept any person applying for basic insurance and cannot differentiate tariff on grounds of health status. Patients can switch health insurers on 1 January every year. In 2006, 18 per cent of people changed their insurer but this had dropped to 6.5 per cent between 2013 and 2014.[3] Besides a basic health insurance package, patients can choose to buy complementary policies with any insurer but insurers are not obliged to take them.

While the fall in the number of people switching insurance companies is a worry, the industry appears to remain competitive with consumer choice an effective force. In health services more broadly, patient and consumer centricity of is one of the most notable achievements of the Dutch. For the last three years the Netherlands has topped the EuroHealth Consumer Index, which scores countries on a broad range of indicators such as patients' legal rights, accessibility and choice of services, waiting times, provision of quality information (including patient medical records) and health outcomes.[4] Given the competition of nearby Nordic countries and others for this title, it is an achievement of which the Netherlands is rightly proud.

Careful System Design

The Dutch system is carefully designed, with the roles and responsibilities for insurers, providers and government largely well defined and complementary. The Dutch Health Care Authority has primary responsibility for ensuring that markets function properly while the Dutch Competition Authority enforces fair competition between insurers and providers, all subject to the Dutch Competition Act. Alongside these players sit various quality agencies. Care quality is supported through legislation governing professional standards, quality in healthcare institutions, patients' rights and new health technologies. The Dutch Health Care Inspectorate (IGZ) is responsible for monitoring quality and safety. That said, most quality assurance is carried out by providers while professional regulation is based on revalidation for specialist staff and compulsory continuous medical education. On-site peer assessments are organised by professional bodies coupled with organisational accreditation and certification. This information is not always shared with the insurers and others, but things are slowly changing for the better.

There are impressive national quality-improvement programmes based on the 'breakthrough' method 'sneller, beter' (faster, better), which was introduced more than a decade ago, and in 2014 the National Health Care Institute (Zorginstituut Nederland) was established to drive quality, safety and efficiency. Outcomes are good; life expectancy in the Netherlands, at 81.1 years,[5] is just over the OECD average. Smoking and obesity are both below average.

Dutch healthcare reform should command interest and a degree of admiration for a number of reasons. First, the 2006 reforms were aimed at enhancing the principle of social solidarity, not reducing it. Second, although the policy gestation period was more than two decades, a broad-based consensus on the need for reform developed. Third, unlike some government reform programmes elsewhere, the goal of reform was clear and simple: to improve access, quality and efficiency, all stimulated by competition.

Unlike the pattern in some other European countries, once the 2006 reforms were executed they were given time to settle in. Politicians have generally avoided micromanagement, continually adjusting laws or tampering with structures every time a problem has arisen. It remains to be seen whether this hands-off approach will survive the fallout from the economic crisis, which has made health a contentious issue again.

Growing Cost Pressures

While the direction of reform in the Netherlands is clear, it is still a little early to pronounce on its success. It is certainly true that, by international standards, the Dutch health system performs well and public satisfaction is high. It is also true, however, that with 12.4 per cent of GDP committed to health and care services, the Netherlands is now the highest spender in Europe in proportion to the size of their economy.[6] Financial pressures are growing rapidly, and with such a high starting point the Netherlands cannot spend its way out of trouble as its government seeks to cut the budget deficit to below 3 per cent of GDP, the level required across the eurozone.

A recent Dutch Health Care Performance Report provided indisputable evidence that the quality and cost of healthcare across the Netherlands vary substantially between providers. Cost differences of two or three times are not uncommon. Examples of quality variation include large differences in maternity services. The true mettle of the reforms will now be tested; it is relatively easy for the system to accept competition while healthcare spending is growing but an altogether different matter when budgets are contracting.

The pressures in the system were recently exposed in a major political row, which came close to bringing down the government, over whether patients should have free choice over doctors or whether insurers should have the right to send patients only to contracted providers. Currently, patients will be reimbursed for 75 per cent of the cost if they visit a provider that is not contracted. Still unresolved at the time of writing, the dispute is important in determining the balance of power between insurers and patients. Patient choice is clearly an important consideration but the ability of payers to reshape the system will be undermined if they lose the ability to contract selectively.

Unsustainable Hospitals

Talking to major health insurers and providers in the Netherlands reveals a private recognition that many of the small hospitals are unsustainable – notably in rural areas – and some are delivering poor-quality care. The insurers have set about reducing this variation through assertive price negotiation, clinical redesign at scale and changing patient flows, but no one seems to have developed sufficient critical mass to command change and consolidate care. Ironically, insurers feel they are too small while the larger teaching hospitals think the insurers cannot collaborate sufficiently to channel care into the right settings, which builds in inefficiencies. Despite growing evidence of quality variations, the Dutch, like everyone else in Europe, treasure their local hospitals.

There has been a marked trend towards consolidation among the insurance providers, with the number of players falling from 57 in 2006 to fewer than nine in

2015, with the four largest accounting for 90 per cent of total market share.[7] This is leading to concerns about a lack of choice. One mooted solution is to open up the market to foreign companies.

Since the competition-driven system was introduced, the increasing financial pressure facing hospitals – mainly not-for-profit organisations run by charities and religious orders – has led nearly half the hospitals in the Netherlands to declare that they will join forces to form a new insurance plan that will 'see off' policies from the existing insurers to close some hospital sites. It remains to be seen how the Dutch Competition Authority will react to hospital poachers turning gamekeeper, and uptake at present is low.

The insurers are ambivalent about hospital consolidation. They do not want hospital organisations to become too big to fail, nor dominate local markets. Difficulties in the relationship between hospitals and insurers are exacerbated by the contracts being annual, on the grounds that citizens can change their insurer every year; this discourages long-term planning.

In a move which is mirrored in other European countries, Bismarck-type social health insurance allows for voluntary extra insurance or increased patient co-payments or deductibles. The financial crisis has driven many governments with health insurance systems to increase premiums or out-of-pocket payments and the Netherlands is no different. In a heated parliamentary debate, legislation was passed that has led to the obligatory patient deductible excess increasing from €220 in 2012 to €375 in 2015.

Every Dutch person is required to register with a GP, who acts as both navigator and gatekeeper for the health system. They are expected to control costs by limiting specialist referrals. Insurers fund primary care through a capitation fee for patients on their list – around two-thirds of practice income – and a fee for service. In recent years there has been a rapid consolidation in primary care, with solo GPs forming group practices and multidisciplinary health centres, and a much greater emphasis on teamwork.

Tensions with Insurers

While Dutch primary care is rightly the envy of many other nations, an increasingly tense relationship between insurers and GPs is developing. In March 2015, more than half of GPs signed the Manifesto of the Concerned GP, a document protesting against increasing bureaucracy, limitations on prescribing and referral behaviour, and the lack of bargaining power they have under Dutch competition law, which restricts collaboration in their negotiations with insurers over contract terms. Although the insurers may be tempted to enforce their increased purchasing power further, it is crucial that relationships improve soon as strengthening primary care is a core plank of their strategy to focus more on prevention and self-management of chronic conditions.

So far, the extent to which the reforms have encouraged a greater focus on prevention has been disappointing; it appears that insurers are reluctant to invest in long-term health benefits when patients may move to a competitor. With little indication that the reforms are having a significant impact on costs, issues such as waste in the health system are attracting political attention again.

In one of the boldest moves yet to contain costs, in January 2015 the government devolved responsibility for long-term care to the 392 municipalities, simultaneously cutting the overall budget. Old-age care has been a major source of recent cost inflation, and with the ratio of working-age people to people over 67 set to change from 6.5:1 in 2010 to 3:1 in 2030, long-term care is seen as a major threat to the sustainability of the system. The path of reform is risky, however. There is no guarantee that the small-scale municipalities will have the capability to take on this role, especially as devolution has led to a complex web of contracts because the catchment areas of providers rarely align with local administrative boundaries. Long-term care is in for several years of painful upheaval, and it is as yet unclear if the outcome will be worth the effort.

Conclusion

In many ways, the Netherlands is an archetype of the Bismarckian healthcare models of northern Europe. Quality is high and it has achieved a remarkably balanced distribution of power and control. It has yet to find an effective way of dampening the alarming rate of cost inflation, but the blended approach of social solidarity and private sector competition, with government setting the rules of the game, is a fascinating experiment from which other countries have much to learn, both good and bad.

References

1 Commonwealth Fund, Mirror mirror on the wall: How the performance of the US health-care system performs internationally – 2010 Update (Commonwealth Fund, New York, 2010).

2 Health Consumer Powerhouse, Euro Health Consumer Index 2014 (HCP, 2014).

3 Figures from KPMG in the Netherlands.

4 Health Consumer Powerhouse, Euro Health Consumer Index 2014 (HCP, 2014).

5 World Bank statistics, Life expectancy at birth (World Bank, 2012).

6 World Bank statistics, Total health expenditure (% of GDP) (World Bank, 2012).

7 Civitas, Healthcare systems: The Netherlands (Civitas, 2013).

17 Germany
Doctor knows best

Germany created the first social insurance funds for medical care in the world. In 1883 Chancellor Otto von Bismarck established 'sickness funds' which, over time, were expanded to create a universal healthcare system. The founding principles of the system – solidarity, subsidiarity and corporatism – define the quintessential characteristics of German healthcare today. The strength of these principles pose significant challenges for healthcare reform, especially when doctors are regimented into different care silos and seek to preserve payments systems that are buckling under the pressure of an ageing population which needs better care pathways.

It is worth understanding the principles supporting the German statutory health insurance (SHI) system a little more as, like all countries, the culture and traditions of the country are woven into the fabric of healthcare. Since 2009, health insurance has been mandatory through either SHI or private health insurance. SHI covers 85 per cent of the population.[1]

Germans are proud of their universal health system and point to a strong tradition of solidarity dating back to the period of national unification in the nineteenth century. In many countries the principle of solidarity is guarded by the state. While this is also true in Germany, there is much more active participation (and contribution) from employers and staff. Statutory sickness funds are financed predominately through payroll taxes which are currently fixed at 14.6 per cent, split 50/50 between employer and employee.

States in Control

Equally, the principle of subsidiarity was enshrined in the German constitution in the Basic Law of 1949. Germany has a highly decentralised political and administrative system where 16 states (Bundesländer) are largely responsible for healthcare while the federal government plays – and this is a generalisation – more of a regulatory and supervisory role. Subsidiarity in healthcare means the federal and state governments delegate powers to membership-based, self-regulated organisations of payers, providers and physician associations known as 'corporatist bodies'. Participation in the scheme is mandatory.

Corporatism is active in healthcare, with democratically elected representatives from employers and employees participating in the governing boards of sickness funds and other decision-making bodies. This collaboration is designed to make it difficult for any one group to change the rules without the consent of other players. This works when times are good but when there are economic, social or demographic pressures the system can become rigid and protectionist.

Over 130 sickness funds collect contributions and transfer these to the Central Reallocation Pool which, in turn, pays over 2,000 hospitals as well as doctors in ambulatory and primary care. These payment systems reflect the way doctors are organised and, as we shall see, are now frustrating sensible reforms for a sustainable health system.

Hospitals are funded through dual financing, with states paying for capital and sickness funds for revenue. Payment of ambulatory and primary care physicians by the SHI is made from a morbidity-adjusted capitation budget paid by the sickness funds to the regional associations of SHI physicians, which then distribute payments to their members for the volume of services provided. It is important to note that most hospitals are not allowed to see 'outpatients' as these patients are cared for in primary and ambulatory care – an historic division that impedes the development of new, integrated models, albeit that some doctors work across the boundary. Roughly 46 per cent of doctors in the community are family physicians and 54 per cent are specialists,[2] some working in small units and others in larger primary care centres.

The Medical-Industrial Complex

The complexity and decentralisation of the German system make change difficult. Healthcare in Germany is high profile and big business. It provides 11 per cent of all employment (4.9 million people among a population of 81 million) and accounts for over €330 billion of the economy.[3] Over 2,000 hospitals (with roughly a third each provided by the public, not-for-profit and private sectors) with 132 sickness funds and a variety of physician organisations make this 'medical-industrial complex' difficult to reform. It has been suggested that if doctors spent as much time improving quality as they did negotiating reimbursement rates there would be a massive reduction in clinical variation and fewer adverse incidents.

In his book *Network Medicine*, the German tycoon Eugen Münch says that the traditional structures and systems in healthcare have to be transformed.[4] He argues for massive consolidation and integration between the country's hospital providers, community physicians and sickness funds to create large national chains that preserve universal healthcare but integrate to provide German-style accountable care organisations. He notes the paradox that German healthcare has both an acute scarcity of resources and a huge resource inefficiency which will only get worse as the population ages and there are fewer tax-paying workers to support the growing disease burden.

Münch calls for a nationwide hospital network with integrated ambulatory and outpatient care with one or more sickness funds that have the scale, scope and specialisation required to meet pressing demographic and economic forces. In his view, patients would then be systematically cared for in the most appropriate setting (usually community-based) and supported by extensive e-health and telemedicine. This would all be facilitated by greater personalisation and patient activation. Predictably, the book has provoked conservative forces within the medical profession but these disruptive ideas certainly capture the big issues confronting German healthcare.

It surprised me that, despite being the archetypal Bismarckian system, competition does not appear to be a powerful feature. With the exception of a few expanding hospital chains, the provider market is not especially contested nor is there any great rivalry between the sickness funds. Given that private insurance does not appear to be offering much challenge (with a stable share of about 12 per cent of the population covered[5]) it is easy to see why there is increasing debate about the need to encourage greater activism among payers. Structural changes have periodically sought to contain costs in the hospital sector but without any great sophistication or focus on quality. The creation of the Institute for Quality and Efficiency in Healthcare in 2004 was a positive step; it has offered useful system leadership and made Germany one of the most price-competitive pharmaceutical markets in the world but so far it has not created the disruption among payers and providers that many believe the system needs. A new Institute for Quality is planned for 2015.

Germany has tried to boost the power of patients through the General Law on Patients' Rights, which came into force in 2013. It incorporates into the Civil Code rights and duties around the relationship between providers and patients.

Germany has to face the opportunities and pressures presented by its ageing population. With the world's lowest birth rate and high life expectancy of 81 years, it is projected that by 2019 more than 23 per cent of German citizens will be aged over 65, placing the country second only to Japan in this demographic.[6] Healthcare GDP spend has been increasing steadily and now stands at 11.3 per cent.[7]

Progress on Elderly Care

Reform of the elderly care system has been a priority for government and – with less bureaucratic complexity than healthcare – progress is being made. In January 2015 the First Act to Strengthen Long-term Care (Erstes Pflegestärkungsgesetz) came into effect. Important changes include around €2.5 billion more in residential and non-residential benefits, and better staffing ratios in care homes (from 1:24 to 1:20). The Act also strengthens Germany's generous support for carers, who patients can pay instead of professional home-care staff. This is a novel way of addressing workforce shortages in the sector and has been improved further by guaranteeing 10 days' paid leave if care needs to be arranged for a relative at short notice, such as after a stroke. A further phase of legislation for long-term care is expected in 2017.

If Germany's elderly care financing points the way for other countries, its payments for primary care offer a cautionary tale. In 2004 a €10 quarterly co-payment (the Praxisgebühr) was introduced for patients to see primary care physicians. The scheme lasted eight years before being unanimously scrapped by Parliament – a rare event for the diverse Bundestag. The policy failed to achieve its stated aims: the costs of administration swallowed a large proportion of the money raised and it had no lasting effect on reducing demand apart from a small change among people on low incomes. Damning evaluations of the Praxisgebühr are now frequently cited in other countries whenever GP co-payments are proposed.

Health inequalities between the old East and West Germany have narrowed dramatically since reunification. In 1990 the average West German could expect to live around three years longer than their compatriots in the East but this has closed to just one year for men and no significant difference for women.[8] Greater inequalities now exist within some regions of the former West Germany, with some suggesting it is now more meaningful to talk about a north–south divide when it comes to German health inequalities.

Alongside its ageing population, obesity provides a major challenge. According to OECD figures, 8.9 per cent of the 20+ age group suffered from diabetes in 2010, putting it fourth behind Mexico, the US and Canada.[9]

Aside from the bureaucracy and vested interests, there is another important reason behind the immotility of the German healthcare system: for the most part it delivers effective healthcare, with low waiting times and high patient satisfaction. So far, the public have been willing to accept the expense and complexity to preserve the status quo. Eventually, however, the balance will change as costs and needs continue to increase and other systems overtake Germany in improving quality.

Conclusion

Germans are famously proud of their social solidarity systems, yet for my money it is an American, Michael Porter, who has most succinctly summed up the current state of care in the country: 'Germans receive more care than citizens in many parts of the world, but not necessarily better care or the highest value care. The evidence points to significant room for improvement.' In his 2012 book *Redefining German Healthcare*,[10] Porter proposes a range of major structural changes which were well received at the time but have yet to provoke any practical changes. These included dissolving the divisions between inpatient and outpatient services, introducing mandatory outcomes reporting, and consolidating the provider market to reduce overcapacity and variation.

Porter's prescription matches the developing problems of Germany's healthcare well. Perhaps the reforms he outlines could be described as moving Germany from 'doctor knows best' to a 'patient gets the best' approach. The symptoms hinting at the chronic problems in the healthcare system may only be in the early stages, but swift intervention will provide a much greater chance of success.

References

1 Nadeem E., Health care lessons from Germany (Fraser Institute, May 2014) p. 15.

2 Busse R., Health Systems in Transition: Germany: Health systems review, (European Observatory on Health System and Policies, 2014).

3 Busse R., (2014).

4 Münch E., Netzwerkmedizin: *Ein unternehmerisches Konzept für die altersdominierte Gesundheitsversorgung* (Springer Gabler, Wiesbaden, 2014).

5 Economist Intelligence Unit, Industry Report, Healthcare (EIU, December 2014) p. 6.

6 EIU, (2014), p. 6.

7 World Bank statistics, Total health expenditure (% of GDP) (World Bank, 2013).

8 Kibele E.U.B., Changing patterns: regional mortality differences and the East–West divide in Germany (Demotrends, 15 March 2014).

9 EIU, (2014), p. 13.

10 Porter M. and Guth C., *Redefining German healthcare: Moving to a value-based system* (Springer: Heidelberg, 2012).

18 Switzerland
You get what you pay for

It is good fortune to be one of the eight million people living in Switzerland. A succession of reports by the OECD and the World Economic Forum show Switzerland has some of the happiest, healthiest and most educated people on the planet. With few other natural resources it has consistently invested in its people – measured by health, wellness, education and employment – which alongside one of the best environments in the world for innovation has secured strong economic growth. This fuels a virtuous cycle for further innovation and success.

I have not seen a less distressed health system in all my global travels. While there are problems and some financial pressures, I have met many Swiss health insurance and hospital executives who believe their system is well designed and sustainable, while acknowledging that its quality – something the Swiss are loath to compromise on – means the cost is high.

Switzerland ranked second to the UK in the most recent US-based Commonwealth Fund report on comparative health systems performance,[1] while its life expectancy is one of the highest in the world – 82.7 years, behind Japan, Hong Kong and Iceland.[2] Waiting times are very low, the population is health-conscious and the Swiss Health Observatory can demonstrate excellent outcomes for heart disease, strokes and cancer (although suicides are somewhat high).

In many respects, the Swiss health system is a perfect example of the maxim 'you get what you pay for'. It is the one of the most expensive systems in the world, with health spending representing 11.5 per cent of GDP.[3] Health spending per person, at US$9,276 per annum, is slightly above that of the US.[4] Total healthcare spending is forecast to grow 4–5 per cent a year over the next few years, much higher than Switzerland's anticipated economic growth. This has led some commentators to believe there will be a day of reckoning, although recent political and public discussions suggest the population is not yet prepared for this conversation.

Cantons and Communes

The Swiss health system has been widely examined but, as always, history and cultural context are crucial. Switzerland has a highly decentralised political system through the 26 cantons, with a variety of German, French and Italian first languages. The cantons are largely responsible for the funding, delivery and administration of healthcare, including licensing providers and hospital planning. It is this that drives the fragmentation of the system, with around 300 public and private hospitals serving a population of barely eight million. However, since 2009 the cantons have at least been required to coordinate their planning, which has been further encouraged by the free movement of patients between cantons since 2012.

The federal government oversees regulation while the communes – all 2,596 of them – are responsible for care of the elderly in the community. The highly fragmented nature of the system reflects the country's history and its highly consensual nature, which requires the use of a referendum when more than 100,000 signatures are collected to call a 'popular vote'.

In 1996 the Federal Health Insurance Act mandated that all Swiss citizens were to be individually covered through private not-for-profit health insurance. Individuals are free to choose one of the 67 health insurance operators, which cannot refuse to provide cover. Premiums for a standard package can vary between insurers, age groups and cantons but an insurer may not charge different premiums within a canton to different people within the same age bracket. The insurers can make a profit on supplementary packages. Individuals and families on low income or income support receive health insurance subsidies from the federal and cantonal governments.

So the Swiss model provides universal coverage in an insurance premium-funded system characterised by competition among both insurers and healthcare providers and stimulated by patient choice and high levels of consumer awareness and responsibility. A perfect free-market dream? Not quite.

Since 2012, most of the hospitals are paid by a system based on the case mix (using a Diagnosis-Related Group classification for each treatment) while general practitioners are paid either a fee for service or a bundled/capitation payment if they belong to one of the health maintenance organisations (HMOs). These have been gaining popularity as insurance premiums and co-payments have increased. Prices are set by the cantons.

Government spending on healthcare only amounted to 66 per cent of the total in 2013, much less than the OECD average of 72 per cent,[5] mainly because co-payments are built into the Swiss system of health insurance. These costs have risen substantially even though they are capped, with the Geneva Physicians Association claiming that premiums have increased by 125 per cent over the past 20 years.[6] In addition, some 40 per cent of the population take out supplementary insurance.

Cost-cutting has been a government priority and some insurance premium growth has been reduced through regulation and more widespread use of generic drugs. The problem, say critics, is that the health insurance market together with the large number of small hospitals is too fragmented across the cantons. But progress on reforming the structure and financing is likely to remain slow, held back by public opposition, the size of the cantons and the difficulty of getting legislation approved by referendum. Many cantons show a strong loyalty to 'their' public hospitals while the diagnosis-related payments system is being cross-subsidised to protect local access even though it exposes wide variations in clinical quality and cost.

Voters Back Quality

Over the past decade, attempts to control costs have foundered. Government reforms failed in 2004 while in 2012 a 'managed care' approach to reducing costs was rejected by the electorate on the grounds that care quality could be compromised. In September 2014, 62 per cent of voters in a referendum rejected a plan for a seismic shift from the country's private health insurance system to a state-run scheme,[7] despite evidence that ordinary citizens were feeling the strain of healthcare premiums and co-payments. It is typical of Swiss democracy that they were able to debate the trade-offs between quality and cost in a national referendum. The result is all the more remarkable considering that half the population now belongs to some form of managed care organisation through physicians' networks or HMOs.

Following that vote there is little agreement on how to proceed. Health insurers claim premiums must rise because of an increasing and ageing population, while the government's Health 2020 Strategy suggests savings of up to 20 per cent.[8] It is difficult to find a consensus because there are too many system players with parochial interests. However, there is growing agreement around the need for bundled payments (paying for set treatments for a specific condition), better coordination between clinicians and a greater incentive for patients to adopt cost-conscious care. Until recently, patient empowerment has not been a priority but there is now a greater emphasis on self-management.

The Struggle for Transparency

Switzerland is struggling to identify the right approach to improving quality. The canton structure means national standards for health are elusive and implementation of national health programmes is often poor while local prevention programmes are often effective. Compared with many other developed countries, Switzerland does not have a clear national picture of the standard of its healthcare and lacks a focus on quality and safety improvement. Initiatives are fragmented and dissemination of good practice is slow. One side-effect of the lack of a national picture is that there is relatively little emphasis among politicians and clinicians on health inequalities, although the differences are probably less marked than in many other OECD countries.

Given the sophistication of the Swiss healthcare system and the country's tremendous experience of regulation in the financial services sector, it is surprising that professional self-regulation has been the traditional approach to quality improvement in healthcare. Professionals and providers must be licensed to practise and receive ongoing education for fitness to practise. However, the recently approved Quality Strategy of the Swiss Health System seeks to support hospitals in their performance on acquired infections, surgical safety and medication errors. Professional networks are increasingly emerging, with the encouragement of the cantons, to address areas such as palliative care, dementia and mental health.

Like many other countries, Switzerland needs more health staff. Its medical schools are producing too few graduates, and while an influx of doctors from abroad has helped – around a fifth of clinicians are immigrants – this has distracted the authorities from addressing the problem. Since 2013, restrictions have been imposed on issuing medical practice licences to foreigners in an effort to increase domestic supply.

Conclusion

The challenges Switzerland faces are common to many other countries: the need to give more power to patients, reduce unacceptable variations in outcomes, improve coordination between services and manage costs. But the clear message from its health system is that the best medicine is a thriving economy coupled with a sense of personal responsibility for staying well.

References

1 Commonwealth Fund, Mirror on the wall: How the performance of the US healthcare system performs internationally – 2014 Update (Commonwealth Fund: New York, 2014).

2 World Bank statistics, Life expectancy at birth (World Bank, 2013).

3 World Bank statistics, Total health expenditure (% of GDP) (World Bank, 2013).

4 World Bank statistics, Health expenditure per capita (World Bank, 2013).

5 World Bank, Public health expenditure (% of total health expenditure) (World Bank, 2012).

6 *Sun Daily*, Swiss reject switch from private to state health insurance (*Sun Daily*, 29 September 2014).

7 *Sun Daily*, Swiss reject switch from private to state health insurance (*Sun Daily*, 29 September 2014).

8 Federal Department of Home Affairs, The Federal Council's Health Policy Priorities: Health 2020 (Swiss Confederation, 2013).

19 Italy
No longer 'la dolce vita'

With a profound apology and acute embarrassment, the hotel receptionist in Milan explained that a new tax had been introduced to help the country's beleaguered economy. On a sliding scale, linked to the number of stars the hotel had, guests had to pay the tax per person, per night. She was at pains to explain that the hotel had no control over this and blamed the government.

If only this simple tax could solve Italian debt and lift the pressures off its health system. Fellini's film of 1960, *La dolce vita* (the sweet life), is an image of better days that no longer resonates in Italy as it grapples with chronic fiscal problems and severe austerity measures.

During the early twentieth century, Italy had a social insurance system similar to other European Bismarckian systems. A large number of occupational schemes administered through a variety of independent agencies provided cash benefits and direct medical assistance through contracts with doctors, hospitals and pharmacists. After a fairly tortuous political process the National Health Service (Servizio Sanitario Nazionale, or SSN), styled on William Beveridge's model for the NHS in Britain, was created in 1978 with universal, tax-funded access to healthcare. These services, provided free or for a minimal charge, covered all major needs.

While the SSN was modelled on the NHS as a single, tax-financed payer, a striking difference is the degree of decentralisation and devolution of power to its 20 regions. National legalisation from 1992 to 1993 and constitutional changes in 2001 have radically changed the SSN by giving regions most of the political, administrative and financial responsibility for healthcare. In the current financial crisis, this could have serious consequences.

With a GDP health spend of 9.1 per cent[1] and an average life expectancy of 82.3,[2] the Italian health system is strong by international standards. In 2000, WHO's only World Health Report ranked Italy's system second only to France in its assessment of 191 countries[3] while in 2014 Bloomberg rated Italy third – after Singapore and Hong Kong – in its ranking of healthcare efficiency.[4] Surprisingly, such achievements are rarely mentioned in Italy and are certainly not used to defend the status quo in a way that some French or British commentators do. This may be because a series of patient and public surveys reveal widespread dissatisfaction. Successive Eurobarometer reports point to discontent, especially in the poorer southern regions which historically have had worse services and facilities. Some believe that the increase in regional decentralisation will fuel interregional disparities and undermine the egalitarian principles on which the health service was established.

Local Politics

While the Italian Ministry of Health retains overall responsibility, the regions and local healthcare agencies (LHAs) ensure the delivery of services. Recent reforms create a model in which any provider – public or private – is expected to compete on cost and quality and the LHAs act as commissioners in a quasi-market not unlike the NHS in England. However, at every level the service is subject to local political democratic control and LHA directors are appointed for fixed terms by the regional government. This has significant consequences for the ability to secure reforms.

There is an uneasy stand-off between central government and the regions in the management of healthcare finance and expenditure reduction. Following the eurozone crisis, the government of Mario Monti announced real term funding cuts of €1 billion on a national health budget of around €108 billion. While the percentage is small, this is the first time in the history of the Italian national health service that an absolute reduction in expenditure has been planned and it is far from clear who is taking primary responsibility for making the cuts.

While the regions are responsible for implementing these cuts, they have run substantial deficits for political reasons – in some cases pushing up local taxes – and there is a blame game between political parties nationally and locally. In the past, a tendency by central government to cover regional healthcare deficits undermined incentives to reduce spending and improve efficiency, but this was stopped in 1997 with legislation introducing 'recovery plans'. Given the political patronage and appointment of LHA directors, the system is perfectly designed for protecting the status quo, which frustrates the impetus for clinical and structural reform.

Urgent Need for Reform

The Italian care system is in desperate need of change. With over 650,000 staff, one of the highest doctor/patient ratios in the OECD, and more than 1,000 hospitals serving a population of 61 million,[5] there is overwhelming evidence that the Italian model of care is too hospital centred. With a high beds-to-population ratio by European standards, rationalisation is required so that funds can be reinvested in seriously fragmented primary and community services.

While it would be unfair to suggest that no action has been taken – the number of hospital beds decreased from about 7.2 per 1,000 population in 1990 to 3.4 per 1,000 in 2011[6] – a lot more needs to change. Often the political will and managerial skill is lacking to consolidate hospital facilities and develop a more progressive model of care based on ambulatory services and primary care, which needs to be reorganised to aggregate GPs and provide a more effective network with long-term care services.

Primary care reform has been mixed. Most GPs – who act as gatekeepers to specialists and hospitals – are paid a mixed capitation and fee-for-service rate. Traditionally, many have worked in solo practices but recent legislation is pushing consolidation, such as networks of practices developing common clinical guidelines and electronic records systems. While these improvements are welcome, doctors have resisted change and it has been partially and unevenly implemented, with weaker progress in the south. When this is coupled with the lack of either the resolve or the ability to reduce hospital operating costs and unwarranted clinical variation between hospitals, there is a significant probability that services will not be modernised.

But new regulations since 2007, the recovery plans and new financial reporting procedures for regions, LHAs and hospitals have made the control of money stronger than in the past. This has considerably strengthened the prospects of making the system sustainable but what is still missing is a medium- to long-term vision for the models of care that need to be developed to meet changing patient needs. The urgency of a solution is only compounded by age structure of Italy's population (already one of the oldest in Europe with 21 per cent over 65[7]) and worsening child health (among OECD countries Italy has the least active[8] and second most overweight children[9]).

Getting a Grip on the Money

The recovery plans (piani di rientro) the government has been imposing over the last eight years are making a noticeable difference, with the national government, in effect, overriding the constitutional healthcare powers of some regions. They have significantly reduced deficits and identified improvements in healthcare provision, such as changing the balance between hospitals and community care; these changes must be implemented before the regions can be released from the recovery plan and get their powers back. The plans have a sharp political edge – regional tax rates are automatically raised if deficits are not being covered, meaning there is a high political price for failing to improve the quality and cost of care.

New patient co-payments are appearing. While primary and inpatient care are free at the point of use, co-payments have been applied for ambulatory specialists, imaging and laboratory services, and outpatient drug charges have been levied regionally. Health service staff have been enduring a three-year pay freeze and variations on a vacancy freeze are in place in different regions.

There have been moves towards integrating health and social care, with some regions pushing GPs to work in multidisciplinary teams with specialists, nurses and social workers who together oversee the care needs of the local population with an emphasis on treating people in the community. But again progress is patchy and has proved tough to achieve. This 'medical home' approach (patient-centred, team-based care in the community) is being developed in Emilia-Romagna in the north, where it covers around 700,000 people, and the central region of Tuscany.

Inequalities in health services and outcomes between the prosperous north and the less affluent south is a longstanding problem. Southern regions tend to have poorer community services and worse access to specialist tertiary care, forcing many patients to travel north. Attempts to allocate resources based on need have not made a substantial difference and the allocation of funds between regions remains contentious. While most hospitals are owned by the region, it is notable that in the prosperous northern region of Lombardy almost a third of hospital care comes from the private sector. This region has encouraged competition between public and private hospitals.

The European Commission classifies public sector corruption in Italy as high and this affects healthcare. Problems include prices and payments for drugs and devices, bribes to doctors to skip waiting lists, outsourcing contracts, accreditation of institutions that do not meet minimum standards for safety and quality, and payments to hospitals for the wrong tariff. According to one study: 'The split between the central government responsibility for health financing and the regional responsibility for health expenditure has amplified the problems of accountability in regional health care systems.'[10]

Conclusion

While Italy has shown remarkable resolve in putting its economic house in order and the healthcare recovery plans show a determination to get a grip on costs, the path it has chosen in healthcare is little more than a traditional cost-cutting programme – wage and vacancy freezes and reduced payments for supplies. This will yield some results but it will not keep pace with demands from an ageing population needing different care models. A new political, medical and managerial alliance and compact is needed which will break the current impasse. Italy has a decent health system and deserves to do better.

References

[1] World Bank statistics, Total health expenditure (% of GDP) (World Bank, 2013).

[2] World Bank statistics, Life expectancy at birth (World Bank, 2013).

[3] World Health Organization, The World Health Report 2000 – Health systems: improving performance (World Health Organization: Geneva, 2000).

[4] Bloomberg, Most efficient healthcare 2014: Countries (Bloomberg: New York, 2014).

[5] Economic Intelligence Unit, Healthcare report (EIU, May 2014).

[6] World Bank statistics, Hospital beds (per 1,000 people) (World Bank, 1990 and 2011).

[7] World Bank statistics, Population ages 65 as a percentage of the total population (World Bank, 2013).

[8] OECD, 'Physical activity among children' in Health at a Glance 2013: OECD Indicators (OECD Publishing, 2013).

[9] OECD, Obesity Update – June 2014 (OECD Publishing, 2014).

[10] Lagravinese R. and Paradiso M., Corruption and health expenditure in Italy, *MPRA*, 43215 (11) (2012).

20 Portugal
The price of austerity

Portugal belongs – along with Italy, Ireland, Greece and Spain – to the group of nations that have faced severe economic, political and social uncertainty within the eurozone. The debt crisis has forced each country to take a hard look at what they spend and has raised difficult questions about the principles relating to social solidarity, health funding and provision. For the people of Portugal, questions about their health system strike at the heart of their democracy and sense of national well-being.

The Portuguese health system has its roots in 1946, when the first social security law was enacted. However, it was only after the revolution of 1974 that the restructuring of health services began, a process that culminated in the establishment of the National Health Service (Serviço Nacional de Saúde, or SNS) in 1979. The SNS is considered a major achievement of the democratic government but it is now under pressure after the country was forced to seek assistance from the European Financial Stabilisation Mechanism. This bailout required Portugal to cut spending in all sectors, including the sensitive area of health.

The SNS, which provides universal coverage, is predominantly funded through general taxation. It exists alongside private voluntary insurance but is the largest employer and provider of healthcare. Financial resources dedicated to health consume a relatively high proportion of the country's wealth, but the long-term trend of steady increases in the health budget has seen a dramatic reversal since the global financial crisis. Health spending dropped from 10.8 per cent of GDP in 2009 to 9.7 per cent in 2013,[1] a substantial fall considering that Portugal's overall GDP was also falling during this period. The bulk of cuts have been in the public system, resulting in a shift in the government's share of health spending from 68 per cent to 64 per cent since the recession.[2]

Like many countries that claim to have a universal health system based on the principles of social solidarity, Portugal has a blended system of finance and provision. In addition to the SNS, insurance schemes exist for certain occupations, to which both employers and staff contribute. In addition, around 15 per cent of the population have private health insurance,[3] mainly through corporate group policies. Many of those who buy private health insurance use it as a supplementary service to the SNS rather than a replacement.

Planning and regulation of the health system is overseen by the Ministry of Health and its institutions while the management of the SNS takes place regionally. There are five regional health administrations that are accountable to the ministry for strategic management of population health, supervision and control of hospitals, management of primary care, and the implementation of national policy objectives, including contracting services with private sector providers. The regional administrations pay for primary care but hospital funding is under the jurisdiction of the Ministry of Health.

Performance and Quality

Healthcare regulation is carried out by a number of bodies, the most important of which is the Health Regulation Authority (Entidade Reguladora da Saúde, or ERS) which regulates the activities of all public and private providers. Established in 2003, the ERS is an independent regulator whose principal purpose is to safeguard the interests of service users. Unusually, both the International Monetary Fund (IMF) and the EU insisted that the ERS establish a hospital performance benchmarking system as a condition for financial assistance to Portugal. In response, the ERS has developed the National System of Health Quality Assessment which publishes quality measures based on five dimensions: clinical excellence, patient safety, facilities, patient satisfaction and patient focus. The ERS aims 'to induce an unprecedented change in the way hospital managers, health professionals and healthcare users think about the quality of healthcare in Portugal'.[4]

Other health reforms have affected health promotion, long-term care, primary, ambulatory and inpatient care, and hospital management. Some steps are being taken to improve the coordination of services, including the launch of a long-term integrated care programme, the development of family health units and the increasing use of quality systems. The pharmaceutical industry has been under pressure to cut costs, and access to some drugs has been restricted.

There is a lot to do in ensuring consistent quality. For example, the OECD has revealed wide variations in the rates of healthcare activity in different parts of the country; some areas have double the rates for cardiac procedures as others.[5]

The previous decade of economic growth saw the introduction of new public–private partnerships. In 2002 the government announced a programme for 10 new hospitals using partnerships. These included complicated schemes for building and running four hospitals (Braga, Cascais, Loures and Vila Franca de Xira). Each hospital had two partnerships: the first (InfraCo) was to design, build, finance, maintain and manage the facilities for 30 years with a fixed annual rent while the second scheme (CliniCo) runs the clinical services under a 10-year contract based on production. By international standards it is unusual to have a public–private partnership running clinical services.

With one partnership (construction and management) providing the services to enable the second partnership (clinical) to operate, the contracts are, to say the least, complex, with a consortium of companies involved in running each hospital, one management contract with both integrated and separate parts, and two payment schemes. The partnerships have been controversial, but the clinical partnerships appear to have produced reasonable value for money for the government. They may provide an example for other countries to consider.

Austerity Bites

Despite these changes, many commentators believe that overall reform of the health system has stuttered and been poorly choreographed. Management systems are old-fashioned, with a heavy layer of bureaucracy and political micromanagement. Some believe that it is only through the conditions applied by the EU and the IMF that radical change will take place. This was enshrined into a memorandum of understanding which signalled significant budget cuts and structural reforms to the economy. This included cuts to hospital operating costs and action to eliminate their debts, cuts in spending on pharmaceuticals through tight controls such as the use of generics, massive reductions in health benefits for civil servants such as the police and the military, moves to increase competition among private providers as well as reduce the fees paid to them, and centralised purchasing of medical goods.

Other commitments included better provision of family doctors in all parts of the country, moving staff from hospitals to primary care, developing the role of nurses, and increasing by at least 20 per cent the maximum number of patients per primary care doctor. The government agreed to aim for a reduction of at least €200 million in the operational costs of hospitals in 2012, through cutting and sharing managers, concentrating and rationalising state hospitals and cutting beds.

So Portugal offers a ringside seat for those interested in how austerity and EU intervention affect health systems. Unfortunately, the results have been all too predictable: a loss of healthcare sovereignty driving short-term cost-cutting instead of long-term value creation, a loss of reputation instead of an increase in trust, and increasing co-payments which undermine the founding principles of social solidarity. Minister of Health Paulo Macedo said in 2012: 'This is the budget no minister would like to have', adding that 'we cannot allow uncontrolled spending to continue'.[6] However, in June 2014 Portugal left the European Union Economic Adjustment Programme – the bailout mechanism – and in recent months there have been the first hints of better news.

The Health Price of Economic Collapse

It is one of the cruelties of Portugal's economic collapse that austerity is driving up demand for healthcare just at the moment the country is least able to respond. Most of the population have experienced a reduction in their standard of living, which will have affected overall health and well-being. Problems include poorer nutrition and growing addiction to drugs. Life expectancy has risen steadily and currently stands at around 80 years – above the OECD average but lower than comparable European countries.[7] The sharp drop in living standards could undermine life expectancy progress.

Low productivity in the health sector has plagued Portugal, but painful labour reforms are now taking place. For public health staff used to 14 monthly salary payments (including one extra payment in the summer and another at Christmas) there has been a reduction to 13, along with a 10 per cent cut in wages. As with many European nations, Portuguese law makes redundancy or dismissal for poor performance difficult.

Public healthcare facilities have been closed and public hospitals merged and there are an increasing number of private sector franchise agreements for the management of public facilities in an attempt to overcome weak financial controls which often lead to overspends. The managers of these franchises have significant freedom to control costs, including salaries. Several state-owned hospitals have been turned into public companies, allowing them similar flexibilities. Among all these changes, rural communities fear the loss of their health services.

Conclusion

This financial crisis has caused significant pain for Portugal but in response there has been little strategic debate about the options for a sustainable health system. Instead, a combination of draconian cuts, increased co-payments and reduced entitlements has eroded public confidence. While there has always been some co-payment in Portugal, it has never been described as this within the health service. Now increased user charges are making this 'stealth tax' all too obvious, with charges for consultations, drugs and inpatient admissions.

It is clear that the country and its health service are in transition but the sense of anxiety, size of task and sheer magnitude of the needed economic recovery are blocking out any discussion on vision, values and affordability. The loss of financial sovereignty has cost Portugal control of its own healthcare destiny. Let us hope that recent signs of recovery lead to rejuvenation.

References

[1] World Bank statistics, Total health expenditure (% of GDP) (World Bank, 2013).

[2] World Bank statistics, Public health expenditure (% of total health expenditure) (World Bank, 2013).

[3] Economist Intelligence Unit, Industry Report, Healthcare (EIU, January 2013) p. 5.

[4] Simões J, The Portuguese healthcare system: Successes and challenges (Siemens, 2012).

[5] OECD, Geographic Variations in Health Care: What do we know and what can be done to improve health system performance? (OECD Publishing, 2014).

[6] Augusto, GF, 'Cuts in Portugal's NHS could compromise care' in *The Lancet*, 379 (9814) (2012).

[7] World Bank statistics, Life expectancy at birth (World Bank, 2012).

21 France
Neither Beveridge nor Bismarck but the Republic

To understand France and its public services it is important to understand the nature of the Republic. From Napoleon onwards there has been a degree of indivisibility between the creation of the Republic and the role of the state. Public services are entwined with national pride and a sense of what it is to be French. It has been said that the health system can be explained by the philosophy of national solidarity, based 'around the concepts of both mutual dependence and national obligation'.[1] At its best the sense of state and public service epitomise what is great about French civic rights and responsibilities, but this can produce a degree of insularity which fosters complacency. This certainly applies to healthcare.

Ever since the first (and only) WHO national performance table placed France in pole position in 2000 there has been a sense across the country that the system leads the world.[2] This report is frequently cited as the reason why the status quo must largely be preserved, but in the intervening 15 years (the exercise was not repeated because of doubts about its methodology) many other systems have improved while French healthcare has remained relatively static, notwithstanding limited reforms to hospital financing in 2004. Now the economic crisis is placing great pressure on both national politics and healthcare. France spends 11.7 per cent of its GDP on health, among the highest in Europe,[3] while its per capita expenditure of US$4,864 per annum leaves little room for the country to spend its way out of trouble.[4] In 2014 the French national insurance fund Caisse nationale de l'assurance maladie (CNAM) posted a deficit of over €7 billion, on a budget around €170 billion.[5] Debate on reform has resurfaced but some question whether there is sufficient political will to grasp the nettle.

Carte Vitale and Medecine Liberale

Healthcare in France is characterised by a national programme of social health insurance (NHI), in contrast to the British NHS, which is focused on providing the service itself rather than reimbursing costs. The NHI is managed almost entirely by the state and publicly financed through employee and employer insurance contributions and earmarked taxes. For most patients medical goods and services are not free at the point of delivery but the innovative introduction of the 'carte vitale' (which approximates to a credit card identifying your national health insurance rights) ensures that patients receive the correct level of reimbursement almost immediately afterwards, for example 70 per cent for visiting your GP or 100 per cent for treating specified serious illnesses.

For a system that prides itself on the national principles of social solidarity it is instructive to note that the mandatory NHI only accounts for 77 per cent of total healthcare spending, with the remainder coming from private sources in the form of out-of-pocket payments and private voluntary insurance schemes.[6] The proportion of the population enrolled in a private plan has grown from 50 per cent in 1970[7] to around 90 per cent,[8] as voluntary insurance has increasingly made up for the shortages in NHI funding. With a weak economy and high unemployment this is causing growing public concern. Similar trends can be seen throughout Europe but the distinguishing aspect of the French system is that one major insurer forms the bedrock of the financing system and is then 'topped up' through personal choice.

Although the financing of healthcare still comes predominantly from public sources the provision of healthcare is much more mixed, with about a third of hospitals being for-profit, a fifth not-for-profit and the remainder public, especially the large urban teaching hospitals. Around 40 per cent of France's hospital beds are provided by the private sector (largely for elective care) and patients are free to choose between public and private sector institutions, as this is largely reimbursed through insurance payments.

Patient choice is a strong feature of the system and individuals are free to refer themselves to either a general practitioner or specialist, although a number of reforms are seeking to moderate this and make the GP the gatekeeper. This patient choice – known as the concept of 'medecine liberale' – is a touchstone of the French system and refers to the direct payment made by the patient to the doctor at the point of use, according to the services provided. It is seen as protecting the patient's freedom to choose and a doctor's freedom to practise and prescribe. These three principles – personal payments, choice of doctor and clinical freedom – form the three pillars of French healthcare. However, these pillars are now in danger of being too rigid. The test for French healthcare reform will be to preserve what is good while changing what inhibits integration, cost efficiency and consolidation.

Unlike other parts of Europe, where there is a difference in quality between public and private providers, the French system expects the same level of care. So the system promotes choice over competition – an important, and often misunderstood, aspect of French healthcare. Historically, public hospitals were funded on a block contract and private providers on a fee-for-service. Recent reforms sought to create a common tariff for all providers but there was a political backlash which halted this development because the lower costs in the private sector were placing too much financial pressure on public hospitals. Implementation was abandoned by the socialist government of President François Hollande.

More worrying perhaps is the low pay of doctors and the increasing co-payments for patients to see them. On a recent visit to France it was clear this was an increasing source of anxiety for patients asked to pay out-of-pocket and above-standard rates to see the specialist of their choice. While waiting times for consultations and admissions are low, an increasing number of areas have too few doctors, which is causing political problems. A report of the High Council for the Future of Health Insurance, a permanent body created by the Public Health Act in 2004, found increasing difficulties for patients in these areas trying to get appointments with a doctor who does not practise 'extra billing'.[9]

Good Choice, Weak Coordination

While the system promotes choice it has been less successful at delivering coordination of the different types of care. Primary, secondary and community care are still in silos. In 2009 a major initiative was launched to tackle this by devolving power to new Regional Health Agencies tasked with improving the integration of ambulatory and secondary care and taking a more holistic view of population health. While regional devolution has created structures, it has not created integrated care pathways or people with clear responsibility for integrating the care. This fragmentation and lack of care pathway redesign has worsened inefficiencies and driven up costs. A National Support Agency for the Performance of Health and Medico-Social Facilities (ANAP) has been created to improve benchmarking and introduce improvement methodologies. So agencies are proliferating.

Cost escalation undermines French healthcare performance and is the single biggest threat to its sustainability. Total health spending is in excess of €200 billion but a recurrent deficit of several billion euros has been present for some years. This is being ignored and is storing up problems, especially in the current climate of European austerity.

As well as concerns over co-payments, fraying support for the way healthcare is provided can be seen in growing objections from thousands of business owners and self-employed to paying expensive compulsory health service contributions. This has even ended up in court, with plaintiffs protesting that they should be allowed to sign up with cheaper private insurers rather than be compelled to pay the state.

Serious Inequalities

France suffers from significant and growing health inequalities between regions and social classes, particularly for men. There is a seven-year difference in male life expectancy between the top and bottom social groups.[10] Higher wages have been offered to doctors working in sparsely served rural areas, the government is trying to strengthen rural maternity services and moves have been made to widen access to supplementary insurance by extending eligibility to another one million households.

Reducing health inequalities is one of the aims of a series of reforms aimed at improving public health outlined by the government of President Hollande; these are expected to become law in 2015. Provisions include making every government department accountable for the impact of its policies on public health and health inequalities.

More controversial measures include encouraging the provision of safe injection centres – so-called 'shooting galleries' – for drug users, legal action against those such as student party organisers who encourage excessive drinking and clearer healthy-eating labels for food.

The reforms also aim to improve coordination between services, especially for patients with long-term conditions, and to strengthen primary care. The Regional Health Agencies will be given more flexibility in allocating resources and interpreting national policy. Options include replacing the current fee-for-service model with capitation payments to encourage a greater focus on prevention. The bigger role for primary care is intended to help control the growth of hospital-related spending but it is far from clear whether it will be enough.

In a bold move, in late 2014, the government proposed to scrap user co-payments for primary care, making GP services free at the point of use. The reforms are meeting fierce resistance from clinicians who are concerned about an increase in red tape by the switching of responsibility for claiming reimbursements from patients to doctors. They also argue it will lead to more visits for trivial health problems and have likened the reforms to the imposition of a UK-style NHS.[11] Months of doctors' strikes have ensued and at the time of writing it is unclear who will win the stand-off. With the reforms likely to take many months to refine and implement, little end to the dispute is in sight.

Alcohol consumption has followed the OECD trend in declining, but it is still the highest per capita consumption in the OECD.[12] Alcohol misuse is one of the factors behind an unusually wide gender gap in life expectancy, with women living an average of seven years longer than men.[13] Other causes include a much higher death rate for men on the roads.

France is said to have an 'epidemiological paradox' in that it has low rates of coronary heart disease despite risky behaviours such as high consumption of saturated fat. According to OECD data, France had the lowest mortality rate from ischemic heart disease in Europe – 86 men and 35 women per 100,000; the EU average was 285 men and 167 women.[14] Theories to explain it have been advanced for more than 20 years, covering everything from red wine to the way the government collects the data. Whatever the truth, France is catching up fast on some chronic diseases, with 3.5 million diabetes sufferers – a figure the government predicts to increase by a third in the next five years.

Conclusion

It can be argued that the French system has created an excellent blend of social health insurance, patient choice, professional autonomy, central regulation and a mixed economy of provision which produces good health outcomes. It does not owe its legacy to either Bismarck or Beveridge but to the Republic. However, it cannot afford to deny its deficits for much longer and the health system will have to be better integrated to improve efficiency and effectiveness.

References

1 Wilsford D., *Doctors and the State: The politics of healthcare in France and the United States* (Duke University Press, 1991).

2 World Health Organization, The World Health Report 2000 – Health systems: Improving performance (WHO: Geneva, 2000).

3 World Bank statistics, Total health expenditure (% of GDP) (World Bank, 2013).

4 World Bank statistics, Health expenditure per capita (World Bank, 2013).

5 Economist Intelligence Unit, Industry report: Healthcare – France (EIU, 2015).

6 World Bank figures: Health expenditure, public (% of total health expenditure) (World Bank, 2012).

7 Civitas, Healthcare Systems: France (Civitas, 2013) p. 7.

8 EIU, (2014), p. 4.

9 HCAAM, Rapport annuel du Haut conseil pour l'avenir de l'assurance maladie (HCAAM, Paris, 2006).

10 Commonwealth Fund, International Profiles of Healthcare Systems (Commonwealth Fund, 2011) p. 53.

11 Henry S., French doctors strike in protest at 'NHS-style' reforms (*The Telegraph*, 23 December 2014).

12 OECD, Europe – Health at a Glance 2012 (OECD Publishing, 2012) p. 4.

13 Eurostat figures, Life expectancy at birth (Eurostat, 2012).

14 OECD, Europe – Health at a Glance 2014 (OECD Publishing, 2014).

22 England
The NHS. In place of fear

> This is the biggest single experiment in social service that the world has ever seen.

Aneurin Bevan. 5 July 1948

The National Health Service (NHS) was the first universal healthcare system developed after the Second World War and was founded in 1948 'in place of fear'. After the huge sacrifices of war, people demanded a new settlement across a number of public services and utilities and the NHS was designed to provide free universal care at the point of need, irrespective of age, health, race, religion, social status or the ability to pay. Today in the UK, the NHS is still considered the proudest achievement of modern society and it continues to enjoy popularity and satisfaction ratings greater than those for the Royal Family.[1] It is an iconic symbol of the values of fairness and equity that the people of the UK rightly hold dear.

The NHS Shapes and Saves Lives

Personally, the NHS has both shaped and saved my life and that of my family members as well. Leading the NHS is truly a great privilege and honour. I joined the fast-track NHS Graduate Management Training Scheme over 25 years ago and had the great fortune to be on the Board of Central Middlesex Hospital in my late twenties, lead the University Hospitals Birmingham in my thirties, be the CEO for the NHS region from Oxford to the Isle of Wight and eventually become a Director-General at the Department of Health (in my early forties) and play an active role as a member of the NHS Management Board which was responsible for supporting 1.4 million staff caring for over one million patients every 36 hours.[2] With annual revenues approaching £120 billion, the NHS is responsible for nearly 25 per cent of all public expenditure, a fact that is certainly not lost on the public, patients, practitioners, press, policy-makers and politicians.

At the age of 42, I discovered, quite by chance, that I had prostate cancer. The NHS was magnificent and saved my life. I will spare you the finer details of the radical prostatectomy but my story, in brief, is a quick personal reflection on the NHS. I had superb minimally invasive surgery in a world-famous teaching hospital and was discharged on the same day. The staff were caring, efficient and effective but the integration between hospital and community post-discharge was haphazard, random and uncoordinated. If the technical care I received was at the cutting edge of the early twenty-first century, the communication between the hospital and the community and primary care teams belonged to the late nineteenth century. It was not the fault of any one care professional but the *system* seemed incapable of joining up services to meet my ongoing needs. Similarly, in the case of my mother, now aged 71, the NHS has saved her life on more than one occasion but her multiple co-morbidities and restricted mobility have resulted in 'revolving-door' care as responsibilities have passed between hospital, primary care, community and social services. In spite of these relatively small hiccups, the NHS has always been there for my working-class family and provided care at their time of need without the anxiety of catastrophic financial ruin, bills, invoices or myriad palpitating process steps that can be found in some insurance-based systems across the world. The people of the UK are right to treasure their NHS.

Efficient and Equitable

Indeed, the independent Commonwealth Fund, based in the US, has ranked the NHS as the top health system performer across 11 countries, citing excellent progress in a number of areas.[3] They scored the NHS first in quality, which included effective, safe, coordinated and patient-centred care. Equally, the NHS was ranked first for efficiency and the cost-effectiveness of care and it came second and third respectively for the timeliness and equity of care. As I travel the world, it is bemusing to still correct claims from international healthcare professionals that the UK has very long waiting times and 'death squads' that preside over inhumane rationing. It takes a very long time for performance to change perceptions but the great investments in England's health, not least through the NHS Plan of 2000 to 2008, not only reversed the underinvestment of the three previous decades but put the NHS back on a long-term (if bumpy) trajectory for improved quality, timeliness and responsiveness of care.

Further, the NHS has not been placed outside the top three places in Commonwealth Fund rankings since their reports were established in 2004. While the NHS was ranked only tenth for healthy lives, reflecting issues with proactive care and prevention, the system of universal care has proved to be efficient and effective. At 9.1 per cent of GDP,[4] the UK spends just under the average of OECD countries and enjoys a life expectancy at 81 years,[5] which is on a par with them (although clinical outcomes for certain specialities remain below average). It is a common-held belief that the NHS is funded entirely through progressive taxation but, ever since its inception, the NHS has had a financing blend of general taxation (76 per cent), national insurance or payroll tax (18 per cent) and a small number of co-payments including modest charges for prescriptions.[6] Overall, the NHS is an OECD outlier for the blend of public and private financing of healthcare. According to WHO, general government expenditure accounted for 83.5 per cent of total spending while private sources accounted for 16.5 per cent, resulting in the lowest out-of-pocket costs in the developed world.[7] While approximately 12 per cent of the UK population have private medical insurance, this figure has broadly remained constant through economic periods of boom and bust. Indeed, the average OECD public–private split in expenditure stands at 72 per cent and 28 per cent respectively and it is a largely unremarked fact that the NHS is a lean and efficient tax on business because the drag factor on employers and employees is relatively modest. However, with a low doctor and hospital bed ratio (per 1,000 people) at 2.2 and 2.8 respectively,[8] the NHS will now have to reposition itself to meet the challenges of ageing and non-communicable diseases.

Indeed, it has been suggested that the NHS was one of the greatest British design principles of the twentieth century save the fact that primary care was separated from secondary care and health was separated from social care. Increasingly, through the forces of an ageing population (nearly 20 per cent of the population will be 65 by 2020[9]) and an increase in multiple, chronic conditions (17 million people and rising[10]) health and care need to be better integrated.

In an audacious move just before the 2015 general election, the coalition government, Greater Manchester local authorities and NHS England (the payer and commissioning authority) announced plans to hand over the £6 billion healthcare budget to local control, in what has been termed 'Devo Manc'. The purpose of this was to improve integration, deliver population health gain and increase effectiveness. It is anticipated that devolution will take place by 2017 and it will be fascinating to see whether this democratic accountability will produce superior results.

It is worth noting that the NHS across the UK is no longer one system but four. Since political devolution began in 1999, policy in England, Scotland, Wales and Northern Ireland has increasingly diverged, with England alone pursuing an explicit policy of competition between providers. Outcomes data does not really show any one system clearly outperforming the others but cost per capita in England is lower at £1,912 in 2012/13 (compared to £2,115, £2,109, and £1,954 in Scotland, Northern Ireland and Wales respectively).[11] The rest of this chapter focuses on England.

The Search for Integration

The latest attempt to develop a better strategic integration of health services was announced by NHS England in 2014 with the publication of the Five Year Forward View.[12] Citing the improvements in cancer, cardiac and other clinical outcomes, improved waiting times and patient satisfaction, the Forward View refreshingly laid bare the challenges facing the NHS up to 2020. Left unattended, lifestyle diseases, chronic conditions and ageing will result in a growing demand which 'would produce a mismatch between resources and patient needs of nearly £30 billion a year by 2020/21'.[13] The proposed solutions capture many of the international trends for improved population and public health management, employer-sponsored action programmes, greater patient control of care budgets, more carer support and 'hard-hitting national action on obesity, smoking, alcohol and other major health risks'.

The Forward View also seeks 'to break down the barriers in how care is provided between family doctors and hospitals, between physical and mental health, between health and social care'[14] by better integrating delivery. It is envisaged that new Multispeciality Community Providers (integrated GPs, community, secondary and social services delivering out-of-hospital care) and primary and acute care systems (drawn from examples of accountable care organisations in the US) will form to meet existing and future population challenges.

While refreshing, the Forward View is not without risks. First, it is a perspective and not yet a plan. Second, it assumes that change can be driven through the 200 plus GP-led Clinical Commissioning Groups (an untested and undeclared policy of the coalition government 2010–15) and, third, it makes bracing assumptions that NHS productivity can more than double to 3 per cent per annum by 2020 and release an additional £20 billion of efficiencies on top of flat funding for the previous five years. Even for the most experienced and inspired NHS healthcare leaders, this will be a near heroic challenge. A Stakhanovite call to shovel, no less.

The Forward View also boldly states that: 'In order to support these changes, the national leadership of the NHS will need to act coherently together, and provide meaningful local flexibility in the way payment rules, regulatory requirements and other mechanisms are applied. We will back diverse solutions and local leadership, in place of the distraction of further national structural reorganisation.'[15] This is crucially important for long-term success because the NHS has become world-renowned for rapid policy or structural changes. In all my travels, global audiences often ask three questions: what happened to Connecting for Health (the national IT programme); how can we establish NICE (the National Institute for Health and Care Excellence); and why do you repeatedly reorganise and restructure your health system?

Obsession with New Policies

If health reorganisation was an Olympic sport, the NHS would take the gold medal. Repeated government-instigated reorganisations over the last 40 years expose an unfavourable consequence of politicised medicine. This is something I have given a great deal of thought to over my 26-year experience in healthcare and something I have researched during the writing of this book because I fundamentally believe that success is related to the staying power of leaders, including clinicians. I have also seen a different way of managing in the six years I have led the global healthcare practice at KPMG and this has given me a fresh perspective on traditional wisdoms.

I entered the NHS in September 1989 and during the writing of this book asked my researchers to look at the number of health ministers, Acts of Parliament, national policies and NHS strategic plans that have been announced and launched over that time. While we might quibble over the precise number of national policy initiatives, plans and Acts, the results are Pythonesque. The NHS has enjoyed the leadership of 12 Secretaries of State during this time with a resulting average tenure expectancy of just over two years. Depending on how one counts significant national policy initiatives and laws, the NHS has (conservatively) witnessed 12 in the last 26 years (see box). On top of this the NHS has been rocked by care scandals in the Bristol Royal Infirmary and Mid Staffordshire NHS Foundation Trust (followed by a gargantuan tome from Robert Francis, QC) and seen at least two wide-ranging reports each on health inequalities and long-term aged care. This gives an average policy gestation and birthing period of about two years. Further, in my experience, more energy is spent producing national policies than ever implementing them (with the exception of the NHS Plan which largely stayed the course for eight years).

Major English health reforms: 12 national policy initiatives in 26 years

- Working for Patients (1989)
- Health of the Nation (1991)
- Patients Charter (1991)
- A Service with Ambitions (1996)
- The New NHS: Modern & Dependable (1997)
- The NHS Plan (2000)
- The National Health Service Reform and Health Care Professions Act (2002)
- Choosing Health (2004)
- Our Health, Our Care, Our Say (2006)
- High Quality Care For All (2008)
- Liberating the NHS: Equity and Excellence (2010)
- Five Year Forward View (2014).

No doubt, all these policies made sense at the time (I played a role in four of them) and all had wonderfully motivated protagonists, but the experience detailed in this book shows that long-term, deep-seated sustainable change is largely impossible under such conditions. The NHS has an overactive policy thyroid that needs medication.

Unfortunately, the two-year life expectancy for health ministers and health policy is largely mirrored by the tenure of chief executives within the NHS. As political pressures and justified patient expectations have mounted over the past 15 years, the position of CEO has become both increasingly politicised and problematic, with many now acting more like managing directors than CEOs. The King's Fund recently published a report which revealed that the average tenure of an NHS chief executive stood at just two and a half years and it went on to identify five characteristics of high-performing organisations in the NHS: leadership continuity, a clear improvement methodology, sustained investment in leadership and quality improvement techniques, clear goals and accountabilities, and organisational stability.[16] In his excellent study *The Triumph of Hope Over Experience*, Nigel Edwards looked at the pattern and impact of reorganisation within the NHS.[17] At various stages, politicians have abolished and recreated regional and strategic health authorities from 12 to 8 to 32 to 10 to 0, only to recreate a current pale imitation of four. For strategic commissioning (purchasing) organisations, the position is even worse with a maelstrom of changes mutating district health authorities, primary care groups, primary care trusts and clinical commissioning groups from – respectively – 99 to 304 to 152 to 151 to 221. Interestingly, acute and specialist hospitals have remained pretty constant at roughly 173 throughout the period. Organisational upheaval cannot produce sustainable clinical change and the repeated modifications to commissioning are a serious distraction because general practice (which is widely admired across the world) will need to reform itself as a provider before substantial changes to acute care can meaningfully occur at scale.

New Government

In spite of the pollsters' predictions that the UK general election in May 2015 would be 'the closest in generations', the Conservative Party won an outright majority and, refreshingly, asked Jeremy Hunt to carry on as Secretary of State for Health. This has only been done once before (Norman Fowler 1981 to 1987) and demonstrates the government's desire to promote change through continuity.

Indeed, if Jeremy Hunt's own wish to remain in post until 2017 comes true,[18] he will be one of the most longstanding health ministers in the history of the NHS – only following Norman Fowler and Aneurin Bevan.

At the time of writing, no new policy announcements have been made but the Conservatives pledged in their manifesto and election battle to find an extra

£8 billion of cash towards the £30 billion 'mismatch' identified in the Five Year Forward View – with the balance coming from efficiencies. They also committed to developing 24/7 services to reduce clinical variation (especially at weekends) and extending access to primary care. Pleasingly, they also promised to improve mental health and dementia care although the financial challenge may cast a shadow over some developments. Quietly, commissioning will be allowed to be more promiscuous (as per the Five Year Forward View and 'Devo Manc') and provision more integrated with, paradoxically, more centralised hospital chains emerging.

Strength of Institutions

One of the undoubted strengths of the health service in England is the substantial relationship between academic research and clinical practice. After the publication of High Quality Care for All in 2008, we designated six NHS and university partnerships as Academic Health Science Centres, building on the best practice globally. According to the Times Higher Education World University Rankings, England is home to three of the top five worldwide universities for clinical, pre-clinical and health subjects, and has four universities in the top ten across all subjects: Cambridge, Oxford, Imperial and University College London.[19] In fact, the UK is placed second for hosting the largest number of clinical trials after the US and – in absolute terms – fourth in the world for health research after the US (US$119 billion), Japan (US$18 billion) and Germany (US$13 billion).[20]

Conclusion

KPMG recently brought together 65 global health leaders from 30 countries across six continents to discuss key elements of high-performing health systems. In its report *Staying Power*, the leaders stated that: 'While a restless curiosity for improvement, coupled with an enthusiasm towards innovation, is essential for successful change and adaptation, it's the ability to stay the course that marked out truly exceptional people, performance and progress.'[21] As Jim Collins recounted in his story about Roald Amundsen and Robert Falcon Scott in 1911, success came to the team that were most disciplined and displayed controlled consistency in the most trying circumstances.[22] In fact, the global research carried out by Collins in 'Good to Great' for the corporate sector strongly supports our research in health because he identified that disciplined people, disciplined thought and disciplined action can mark great organisations out from good ones. It's impossible to achieve sustainably high performance if policy and management is changed every couple of years. Thank goodness that clinical and clerical staff usually carry on regardless.

References

[1] Ipsos MORI, State of the Nation 2013 (Ipsos MORI, 2013).

[2] NHS Confederation, Key statistics on the NHS (NHS Confederation, 2015).

[3] Commonwealth Fund, Mirror on the wall: How the performance of the US healthcare system performs internationally – 2014 Update (Commonwealth Fund: New York, 2014).

[4] World Bank statistics, Total health expenditure (% of GDP) (World Bank, 2013).

[5] World Bank statistics, Life expectancy at birth (World Bank, 2013).

[6] Commonwealth Fund, International Profiles of Healthcare Systems (Commonwealth Fund, 2011) p. 38.

[7] World Bank statistics, Public health expenditure (% of total health expenditure) (World Bank, 2012).

[8] OECD Statistics, Hospital bed and physician density, per 1,000 population (OECD, 2012).

[9] House of Commons Library, Population Ageing Statistics: SN/SG/3228 (UK Parliament, 2012).

[10] Department of Health, 10 things you need to know about long term conditions (DH, 2010).

[11] Bevan G. et al., The four health systems of the United Kingdom: How do they compare? (Nuffield Trust, 2014).

[12] NHS England, Five year forward view (NHS England, 2014) p. 5.

[13] NHS England (2014) p. 5.

[14] NHS England (2014) p. 3.

[15] NHS England (2014) p. 4.

[16] Ham C., Reforming the NHS from within (King's Fund, 2014).

[17] Edwards N., The triumph of hope over experience (NHS Confederation, 2010).

[18] West D., Hunt: I want five years as health secretary (Health Service Journal, 26 November 2014).

[19] Times Higher Education, World University Rankings (THE, 2015).

[20] All-Party Parliamentary Group on Global Health, The UK's contribution to health globally: Benefitting the country and the world, (APPG-GH, 2015).

[21] KPMG International, Staying Power (KPMG, 2014).

[22] Collins J., *Good to Great* (Random House Business: London, 2001).

The Americas

23 Canada
At the crossroads

Canadians are rightly proud of their publicly funded health service. Established under the Canada Health Act in 1984, the universal health system is financed through general taxation but organised and run by the provinces and territories. This high level of devolution has deep roots, running back to 1867 when the British North America Act placed healthcare as the provinces' responsibility. Although the entitlements for all Canadians are broadly similar, how those are provided can vary significantly, such that some would argue Canada has not one health system but 13 for the provinces and territories, plus the aboriginal and military systems.

Although the Canadian system defines itself as much by what it is not – American – public funding only accounts for about 70 per cent of total health expenditure.[1] The rest comes from private health insurance, which around two-thirds of Canadians hold to supplement services such as dental, home care and private rooms in hospitals.[2] Service provision is overwhelmingly by the independent sector. The vast majority of physician practices are owned and operated by independent doctors, while hospitals are mostly public or not-for-profit with a few private clinics. Every province except Ontario has adopted a regionalised structure to deliver services, eliminating hospital boards. It is worth noting that fundraising for healthcare and specifically hospitals is an important source of revenue for capital projects and research: in 2013 CAN$1.7 billion (US$1.4 billion, £880 million) was raised from individual donations.[3] There is a very strong and commendable sense of community in most Canadian provinces.

There are striking contrasts in the attitudes and values either side of the Atlantic. In Canada, the health system is fiercely opposed to US-style competition and private insurance, yet Canadians do not seem to feel that personal insurance for home care, 'non-medical services' or rehabilitation represents 'creeping privatisation' – as it would in the UK, for example. Meanwhile, Canadians look anxiously at the gradual introduction of the private sector in providing elective surgery for the NHS. What we tend to see as 'immutable values' around healthcare in different countries often have their roots in historical nudges and fudges in policy and practice.

Indeed, during a recent visit to Ontario – the most populous province – this debate was raging fiercely. The arguments were a mixture of the pragmatic, the professional and the political and reminded me of discussions in the UK just before the introduction of Labour's NHS Plan in 2000, which endorsed the use of private sector treatment centres to clear surgical backlogs and private investment to build new hospitals. Canada is certainly at a crossroads, with tight fiscal constraints now suggesting the need for different policies.

And tough decisions will need to be made. In Ontario for example, the base funding for hospitals has been frozen for the past three years and this is expected to continue. The province has a CAN$10.9 billion budget deficit and the government is trying to squeeze more out of every health dollar. Ontario's health budget currently stands at approximately CAN$50.1 billion and accounts for 42 per cent of all public expenditure. With one of the lowest hospital beds per capita in the OECD, occupancy rates are soaring and hospitals are congested because of a shortage of beds in long-term care and home care. It has been reported that it costs CAN$842 a day to care for a patient in hospital compared to CAN$126 a day for long-term care and CAN$42 for home care.[4] Funding and delivery systems are too wedded to the old hospital and physician fee-for-service model and attempts have been made to confront this.

The Drummond Commission

In a bold initiative the Ontarian government asked an independent and respected economist, Don Drummond, to review the province's long-term finances and make recommendations for public service change. The commission's mandate made clear that he would not be allowed to recommend either higher taxes or privatisation.

While the review took place a few years ago, the commission was extremely well considered and Drummond did not disappoint. Published in 2012, his review was of one of the most comprehensive and high quality I have seen anywhere in the world, and did not pull its punches. Noting that health was the single biggest expenditure item for Ontario, he argued that existing structures and models of care were unsustainable. In words that might resonate across the developed world, he said:

> The public debate in Canada has been poisoned in recent decades by a widespread failure to comprehend the issues or trade-offs that must be made; by knee-jerk reactions to worthy but complex ideas for change; by politicians (and media outlets) who have been too willing to pander to fear-mongering; by stakeholders in the healthcare system who, wishing to cling to the status quo, resist change; and generally by a lack of open-minded acceptance of the reality that change is needed now and that money alone will solve nothing.[5]

Noting that the health system was not in fact a system but rather a series of disjointed services, Drummond's conclusions were similarly bold:

> A shift towards health promotion rather than after-the-problem treatment; a system centred on patients rather than hospitals; more attention to chronic care rather than a primary focus on acute care; co-ordination across a broad continuum of care rather than independent silos; and new ways of dealing with the small minority of patients who require intensive care.

Had his 105 recommendations been acted on, it would have been nothing short of a transformation of Ontario's health system for the twenty-first century: consolidation of hospitals, strengthening of primary and community care, extending the role of nurses, better information technology, outcome-based payment systems, increased home care, investment in prevention, management training in medical schools and a better public–private mix.

But the revolution has not happened. As with so many of these high-level reviews, more attention and effort was put into producing and launching it than implementation. The report suffered from having too many recommendations, but no one ever credibly challenged Drummond's prescription for Ontario's health service. Unfortunately, three years down the line not many of his recommendations have been put into practice.

Greater disruption, however, has been occurring at the national government level in terms of its relationship with the provinces and territories and the distribution of federal funds, which make up around a fifth of healthcare spending. In 2004 the Canada Health Accord was signed, a 10-year plan to boost funding and effectiveness across the country. The Accord guaranteed that federal transfers for healthcare would increase by 6 per cent a year for the next decade, in return for which the provincial and territorial governments would deliver improvements in areas such as waiting times, home care, service integration and the availability of prescription drugs.

Some progress has been made, such as three-quarters of GPs now working in multi-professional practices. In Ontario, doctors are organised into family health teams that have enrolled over one million patients in recent years. Many teams have chosen non fee-for-service payment mechanisms and community health centres with salaried doctors have become more commonplace. Despite this, many more hoped-for improvements have not been delivered. Waiting times are still a problem, there is no effective strategy for prescription drugs and many structural efficiencies remain. I recently spoke at a health conference organised by Queen's University which debated whether there should be a national healthcare strategy for Canada. There was little appetite to swim against the tide and a fairly parochial, provincial perspective prevailed.

Having recognised that fragmentation was a serious problem, most provinces have moved to a regionalised system that ostensibly integrates all services under a single governance structure. However, unlike the systems in Scandinavia or parts of the UK, like Northern Ireland and Scotland, funding and physician payment systems were not reformed and continue to be misaligned. As Steven Lewis notes in the *New England Journal of Medicine*: 'A critical compromise was that physicians remained detached from the regions, which severely restricts the governance and management of clinical practice. It has proved difficult to move substantial funding upstream toward primary and community-based care – a long-standing goal of regionalization.'[6]

Unilateral Government Action

Then, in 2014, the federal government unilaterally overhauled the funding system, saying that future transfers would be based solely on population size rather than healthcare need. This will hit provinces with older or more sparsely distributed populations and could widen the gap between areas such as Alberta, with a young and growing population, and others such as New Brunswick, with a rapidly ageing one.

Central funding is now free of conditions, with the federal government looking to the provincial governments and territories to set their own priorities. This has led to accusations that Ottawa is abdicating its role in shaping healthcare policy. From 2017, the 6 per cent annual increase in federal health transfer will be replaced with a formula linked to economic growth (with a floor of 3 per cent annual increases). Overall, Canada now spends 10.9 per cent of its GDP on health – towards the higher end of OECD countries.[7]

Although the Canada Health Act requires every province to cover a minimum set of treatments under the Medicare system – including all medically necessary care in hospitals and by physicians – there is significant variation in access to healthcare across the country. Provinces vary on whether they cover long-term care, rehabilitation, eye care and mental health, and which groups are eligible for additional entitlements. Perhaps the most significant variation exists in what drugs are available on Medicare (other than for older people and those on low incomes) and what prices the provinces pay for them. There is now some movement among provinces to coordinate their decision-making and purchasing to drive down prices and level up access.

In a study of the healthcare systems of 11 advanced nations, published in 2014, the Commonwealth Fund ranked Canada 10th, just beating the US, with poor scores for safety, timeliness and efficiency.[8] In 2013, Canadians, on average, faced a four-and-a-half-month wait for treatment after referral by a GP; this wait had almost doubled in 20 years.[9] Same-day access to a doctor or nurse is poor compared with many other developed countries and use of emergency services is high.

Disease Burden

The health of Canada's 1.4 million aboriginal people is well below the Canadian average, with higher rates of chronic diseases, infectious diseases, injuries and suicide. The First Nations and Inuit Health Branch of Health Canada, the health arm of the federal government, provides these communities with additional coverage for non-insured health benefits such as prescription drugs, dental and eye care. Recent federal initiatives include the Aboriginal Diabetes Initiative, the

National Aboriginal Youth Suicide Prevention Strategy and the Maternal Child Health Program.

Nationally, heart disease and cancer are the biggest causes of death among the 25 million population. Canada has seen a significant drop in smoking in the last two decades, but the legacy of high smoking rates can be seen in lung cancer death rates relative to other OECD countries, especially among women.[10]

Strong in Research, Education and Telehealth

One area where Canada is leading innovation is in telehealth, partly as a result of the vast distances. The telemedicine network in Ontario is one of the largest in the world, involving all the province's hospitals and many other facilities. It supports clinical care in remote areas, such as access to neurological assessment for stroke patients, which has increased capacity and saved patients from long journeys. A programme for patients with congestive heart failure and COPD has cut emergency and hospital admissions. Psychiatry, paediatrics and dermatology are among other telehealth programmes.

Canada also has a powerful medical and clinical education, research and training platform with a truly international outlook. The Times Higher Education World University Ranking places the University of Toronto, McGill University and McMaster University consistently in the top 20 global institutions based on teaching, research, citations, innovation and global reach.[11] In terms of health outcomes, mortality due to cancer, respiratory and circulatory diseases holds up well against international comparisons and, more locally in Ontario, improvements in waiting times, extended family health teams and community care teams are signs of progress.

Conclusion

The Canadian health system is still revered by its citizens and has many strengths. Its universal access, highly trained professionals and world-class research all highlight the enduring appeal of the Canada Health Act. Nonetheless, the uncertain economic future poses significant questions. There is a political axiom in Canada that you can't win an election on healthcare policy, but you can lose one. Healthcare was barely mentioned in the last federal election and was not a major issue in the last Ontario election in 2014.

Canada's health system, or rather its 13 provincial and territorial health systems, need to find more urgency and resolve for solutions to its healthcare sustainability challenge. A measure of tough love will be needed to maintain enduring values but to change outdated delivery models. Canada stands at the crossroads and needs to find the political will and managerial and clinical skill to establish a progressive coalition of the willing.

References

1 World Bank statistics, Public health expenditure (% of total health expenditure) (World Bank, 2013).

2 Commonwealth Fund, International Profiles of Healthcare Systems (Commonwealth Fund, 2011).

3 Statistics Canada, Volunteering and charitable giving in Canada (Statistics Canada, 2015).

4 Boyle T., Budget will see tough decisions in health, (*The Star*, 22 April 2015).

5 Drummond D., Public services in Canada: A path for sustainability and excellence (Commission on the Reform of Ontario's Public Services, 2012).

6 Lewis S., 'A system in name only – Access, variation and reform in Canada's provinces' in *New England Journal of Medicine* 372 (2015) pp. 497–500.

7 World Bank statistics, Total health expenditure (% of GDP) (World Bank, 2013).

8 Commonwealth Fund, Mirror on the wall: How the performance of the US healthcare system performs internationally – 2014 Update (Commonwealth Fund, 2014).

9 Roy A., If Universal Health Care Is The Goal, Don't Copy Canada (*Forbes*, 13 June 2014).

10 OECD, Health at a glance 2011: Mortality from cancer (OECD, 2011).

11 Times Higher Education World University Rankings (THE, 2015).

24 The US
Let's face the music and dance

The 1936 song by Irving Berlin neatly summarises the paradox facing American healthcare. KPMG research among 200 leading executives across health systems, health plans and life science organisations throughout the US suggests that while everybody can see the need for system change, most organisations are expecting that change to start with someone else. So, while 'there may be trouble ahead' and some people are learning new moves, most organisations are still dancing to the same old tune.

While the scale of change facing China's health system is the largest I have seen across the world, the US's change programme is by far the most complicated. It is sometimes easy to forget that (at 3.7 million square miles) the US is roughly the same geographical size as mainland Europe (3.9 million square miles) and managing change in the US is a little like saying that Europe should have a common, managed healthcare system.

The Urgent Need for Reform

Putting aside the venomous political debate about the Patient Protection and Affordable Care Act (the ACA, or Obamacare), there can be no doubt that serious reform of the country's health system is required. There are a number of compelling reasons to change. America has an estimated national debt of US$18 trillion[1] and currently spends over 17.1 per cent of its GDP on healthcare,[2] delivering a modest life expectancy of 78.9 years,[3] one and a half years less than the OECD average of 80.2 years. On current projections, health spending is forecast to exceed 20 per cent of GDP by 2023, prompting some commentators to wonder whether national security would be compromised if healthcare continued to consume such a high proportion of spending. It is estimated that without reform by 2025 expenditure on Medicare (for older citizens), Medicaid (for poorer citizens), social security and interest debt could consume all federal tax receipts.[4]

Prior to the implementation of the ACA it was estimated that roughly 50 million of the 315 million residents in the US were uninsured.[5] While the Supreme Court ruling of June 2012 upheld the Act (although it struck down the mandate that individual states must add people to Medicaid, the health safety net) and it is now estimated that an additional 16 million Americans have taken up insurance,[6] approximately 20 million people will still be left without cover even when the Act is fully implemented.[7] The OECD estimates that the US government accounts for 46 per cent of total health spending[8] (ironically, a similar level to that of Communist China), which is much lower than the average of most developed countries at around 72 per cent. America spends more on healthcare than any other country in the world but it is the only developed nation that has less than 95 per cent of its people covered by some form of insurance. It has been estimated that 35 per cent of Americans have faced financial difficulties because of medical costs.[9] Moreover, roughly half the population has health insurance which is tied to their job, restricting labour mobility.[10] Rising premiums also come out of wages and healthcare inflation has been cited as one of the main reasons why pay for the average American has stagnated over the past couple of decades.

The excessive costs of the system are well understood; in 2011, the respected Institute of Medicine estimated that US$765 billion a year was potentially wasted through unnecessary and inefficient services, excessive prices and administrative costs, fraud and abuse, and missed opportunities for prevention – almost a third of total health spending.[11] Administrative costs in America are huge – of the order of US$360 billion a year – because of the large transaction costs associated with a multiplicity of payers and providers who still overwhelmingly pay on a fee-for-service basis rather than on value. While the ACA has heralded new forms of accountable care organisations (ACOs), fewer than 20 per cent of all contracts currently reflect this innovative development.

Factors that drive up US healthcare costs include prescription drugs – the country spends roughly double the OECD average per head on pharmaceuticals[12] – plus the fact that US physicians are the highest paid in the world. Research by Medscape in 2014 revealed that a typical hospital doctor earned US$262,000 a year.[13] The Commonwealth Fund consistently ranks the US healthcare system last in studies of major industrialised nations because of its poor access and care coordination.[14] For example, one in five elderly patients discharged from hospital is re-admitted within 30 days.[15] The ACA seeks to redress many of these features but one of the major concerns is that it dramatically increases access to healthcare without making the system significantly more efficient.

Obamacare Makes Progress

Some believe that the extra costs of the ACA do not match the benefits and argue that the business case for implementation was high on hope but low on due diligence. I tend not to agree. As noted, the change programme is complicated and the rollout for implementation is long, with many interdependent factors requiring near-simultaneous change. But early assessments are encouraging. Blumenthal and Collins suggest that, after a shaky start, the marketplaces are now functioning and people have enrolled in new marketplace schemes and Medicaid[16] – 16 million Americans have taken up new insurance cover. Fewer people are uninsured and underinsured and a recent Commonwealth Fund tracking survey estimated that 60 per cent of people that had new coverage had used it while 62 per cent reported that they would not have been able to access or afford this care previously. While encouraging, they also state that 'in some cases, such as cost and quality indicators, drawing a clear causal connection between changes in health system performance and the ACA is difficult'.

This quote strikes at a fundamentally important aspect of the Act. The new law, signed in 2010, wanted to make care more affordable and protect patients. While political debate concentrated on the rights and wrongs of government-mandated, compulsory insurance cover (for example, the July 2015 Supreme Court ruling upholding federal tax credits for citizens living in States without their own exchanges), the existential question is healthcare sustainability. In this respect, the ability of the Act to encourage alternative ways of paying for healthcare as well as finding new ways of organising providers to deliver coordinated care will be mission critical.

I have engaged with many healthcare executives and organisations across America and there are broadly two competing narratives in play. Both have a chance of dominating the future healthcare landscape. The first argument suggests that the ACA has responded to the needs of the country, businesses and citizens and is shaping, through its dominant position as a payer (Medicare and Medicaid), the insurance marketplace and pattern of provision. Healthcare costs are now growing at a much slower rate, with five consecutive years of spending growth just below 4 per cent.[17] Spending over the next decade is expected to increase at a rate of 5.7 per cent compared with 7.2 per cent annual growth from 1990 to 2008 before the ACA was passed.[18]

Proponents of the counter-argument suggest that the global financial crisis and the crippling pressure on employers have put downward pressure on healthcare cost inflation and added vigour and rigour into healthcare reformation. Supporters of this view suggest that change has been very slow, uptake of coverage modest and cost reduction virtually non-existent. They claim that with economic growth now returning to the US, providers will regroup, consolidate, acquire more market power and push up prices. In short, reform will be reversed and business as usual will continue.

Irreversible Change

Whichever of these two arguments is correct (more than likely it is both), real change is now sweeping American healthcare in ways more fundamental than opponents of the ACA could ever reverse. There has been an enthusiastic take-up of ACO-type arrangements, with fee-for-service contracts being replaced by flat-fee payments that incentivise quality, appropriate treatment and cost containment. A target has been set for 50 per cent of Medicare payments to be value-based by 2018, with private payers aiming for 75 per cent by 2020.[19] A quiet retail revolution is also taking place, with retailers and pharmacy chains starting hundreds of new walk-in clinics. These offer quick service, clear pricing and lower costs, capitalising on the increasing deductibles by insurance companies that Americans are having to pay. Between 2007 and 2015 CVS Health started almost 1,000 new retail clinics, Walgreens 400, and Walmart, Target and Kroger several hundred more.[20]

In the *New England Journal of Medicine*, McWilliams et al. have shown how Medicare ACO programmes seem to improve patient experience, citing two important measures: timely access to care and primary care physicians being better informed about specialist care provided to their patients.[21] Further, the Blue Cross Blue Shield of Massachusetts Alternative Quality Contract, which includes approximately 85 per cent of physicians in their network, reports costs savings in the range of 5.8 per cent to 9.1 per cent,[22] while recent reports from the Centers for Medicare and Medicaid Services (the federal agency which oversees the two programmes) suggest that ACOs in the centre's programmes are achieving modest savings and have improved both quality and patient experience measures.

I take encouragement from examples such as Montefiore in the Bronx. This hard-working health system in a tough part of New York was one of the original 32 pioneer ACOs selected in 2011 and the most financially successful. I have met its leaders and clinicians and seen first-hand the challenges of serving a deprived area of the city. As the largest healthcare provider in the Bronx, the poorest urban county in the US, a new ACO has been created which aims to keep people as healthy as possible and out of hospital. In addition to telemonitoring, the ACO provides patient self-education and group classes, home visits and post-discharge outreach palliative care and the coordination of primary care providers, pharmacists and social workers. For their sickest 30,000 patients, Montefiore carried out utilisation reviews and redesigned care pathways and plans accordingly, achieving good results.[23] For example, diabetes admissions have declined by 14 per cent and costs have been reduced by 12 per cent. For health systems like these, there is no turning back.

A lot of policy and the reform programme have tended to concentrate on the technocratic and transactional aspects of change such as organisational structures and payments systems, but less focus has been given to the cultural shifts that are vital if changes are to be sustainable. There is no doubt in my mind that reform is on the move in both for-profit and not-for-profit organisations. But it may not be enough. Mindsets and culture could still derail progress, while the high degree of fragmentation and sheer scale and complexity of the task is exceptionally challenging.

Who Will Lead the Transformation?

In 2012, KPMG researched the views and attitudes of senior executives across health providers, health plans and life science (pharmaceutical and biotechnology) organisations across America. The results, published in *Transforming Healthcare: From Volume to Value*, reveal a paradox.[24] While respondents expected significant change to occur in the health sector over the next five years, they felt their own organisations had 'sustainable or somewhat sustainable' business models. Almost all hospital providers believed moderate or major change was on its way in the next five years while 94 per cent of health plans felt the same. Notably, 87 per cent of life science respondents felt change would happen but only a quarter thought this would be 'major'. This may betray a slight disconnect from the day-to-day pressures and is certainly a far cry from Europe, where some indebted countries have delayed drug payments by up to two years.

All respondents felt the healthcare sector had to integrate services and move from volume to value (the latter broadly defined as the delivery of patient outcomes and quality divided by the costs of the service) because US healthcare was unsustainable in its current form. But there was a significant disconnect between the parties about how it should, and could, transform. While people could imagine a different future, it was abstract and far removed from their current operation.

When providers were asked how they were preparing for the major changes envisaged, 86 per cent thought they would have to manage their cost structure in order to break even on Medicare prices. Around half the hospitals thought this would mean reducing costs by between 11 per cent and 20 per cent – an unprecedented decrease across the industry. When asked how they would meet this pressure, however, 82 per cent of respondents felt they could continue to increase commercial rates (for example, employers, health plans and self-pay schemes) because 'the organisation has enough market power or compelling value propositions to ensure commercial reimbursement rates'.

These beliefs contrast sharply with health plans, where half of respondents forecast a reduction in employer insurance costs. The health plans felt that growth would come from Medicaid and Medicare, so lower cost models would need to be established. Health plans believe employers will demand lower cost offerings and rely on wellness programmes to support this move. Some employers may simply abdicate responsibility for health insurance to their employees, thus creating a retail market with stronger consumer power.

So there are conflicting views, but most industry players expect costs to reduce. It has not been done before and certainly not on this scale. The experience of the UK demonstrates just how hard it is to reduce costs and improve productivity. As an executive from the Johns Hopkins Hospital and Health System, quoted in the *Huffington Post*, put it: 'If you haven't already done a lot of that, you're really going to be behind the eight ball'.[25]

In a predictable development, the need for cost reductions has initiated more provider consolidation, with Brendan Buck, former press secretary to the Speaker of the US House of Representatives John Boehner, claiming 'consolidation promises greater efficiency, but all that ever materialises is greater costs.'[26] More recently, the National Academy of Social Insurance claimed that 'there is growing evidence that hospital–physician integration has raised physician costs, hospital prices and per capita medical care spending'[27] and suggested a similar trend in hospital health plan integration. Many providers would argue, however, that this activity is a forerunner to creating new care models that will do exactly the opposite.

Conclusion

Like many things in the US, fact, opinion and prejudice are hotly debated. No one really knows how the ACA will alter the access, cost and quality balance in American healthcare, but this is a serious attempt and the clock cannot be turned back. My heart is willing it to succeed because my head tells me there will not be so much political capital spent on it again for another generation.

References

1 http://www.usdebtclock.org/.

2 World Bank Statistics, Total health expenditure (% of GDP) (World Bank, 2013).

3 World Bank Statistics, Life expectancy at birth (World Bank, 2013).

4 National Commission on Fiscal Responsibility and Reform, The moment of truth (White House, 2010).

5 US Census Bureau, Health Insurance Highlights 2012 (US Census Bureau, 2012).

6 Bernstein L., Affordable Care Act adds 16.4 million to health insurance rolls (*Washington Post*, 15 March 2015).

7 Congressional Budget Office, Effects of the Affordable Care Act on health insurance coverage: March 2015 Update (CBO, March 2015).

8 World Bank Statistics, Public health expenditure (% of total health expenditure) (World Bank, 2012).

9 The Commonwealth Fund, The rise in health care coverage and affordability since health reform took effect (The Commonwealth Fund, 2015), p. 5.

10 Congressional Budget Office, Effects of the Affordable Care Act on health insurance coverage: March 2015 Update (CBO, March 2015).

11 Institute of Medicine, The healthcare imperative: Lowering costs and improving outcomes (IOM, 2011).

12 OECD Statistics, Pharmaceutical expenditure per capita (OECD, 2012).

13 Medscape, Physician compensation report 2014 (Medscape, 2014).

14 Commonwealth Fund, Mirror on the wall: How the performance of the US healthcare system performs internationally – 2014 Update (Commonwealth Fund: New York, 2014).

15 Robert Wood Johnson Foundation, The revolving door: a report on US hospital readmissions (RWJF, 2013).

16 Blumenthal D. and Collins S., Assessing the Affordable Care Act: The record to date (Commonwealth Fund Blogs, 26 September 2014).

17 Hartman M. et al., National Health Spending in 2013: Growth slows, remains in step with the overall economy, in *Health Affairs,* 10 (1377) (December 2014).

18 Blumenthal D. and Collins S., Assessing the Affordable Care Act: The record to date (Commonwealth Fund Blogs, 26 September 2014).

19 *The Economist*, Shock treatment (*The Economist*, 7 March 2015).

20 *The Economist* (2015).

21 McWilliams J.M., et al., Changes in patients' experiences in Medicare Accountable Care Organizations in *New England Journal of Medicine*, 371, 1715-24 (2014).

22 Song Z. et al., 'Changes in health care spending and quality four years into global payment' in *New England Journal of Medicine*, 371 (18) 1704-14 (2014).

23 KPMG International, Pathways to population health (KPMG, 2015).

24 KPMG International, Transforming healthcare: From volume to value (KPMG, 2012).

25 Young J., Prognosis unclear (*Huffington Post*, 8 October 2012).

26 Japsen B., Insurers fight hospital mergers as ACA snubs fee for service medicine (*Forbes*, 14 September 2014).

27 Goldsmith J. et al., Integrated delivery networks: In search of benefits and market effects (National Academy of Social Insurance, 2015).

25 Mexico
Unfinished business

Mexico is a developing country with big ambitions for healthcare which needs to overcome a serious burden of chronic disease and huge disparities in wealth and access to treatment. It is in the early years of its second major wave of healthcare reforms this century. There are encouraging signs of progress but the obstacles are formidable for the 122 million people of Mexico.

The bold strides Mexico has made towards universal health coverage over the last decade are impressive, enrolling millions of uninsured and underinsured citizens into a new public insurance scheme. The challenge now is making that coverage count in terms of better health services and improved outcomes.

Mexico currently spends 6.2 per cent of its GDP on healthcare,[1] one of the lowest rates in the OECD. Government spending accounts for just half of this, with the other half mostly made up of out-of-pocket expenditure (barely 4 per cent of Mexicans have private insurance).[2] Funding for health is expected to rise rapidly in the coming years, however, with 8.1 per cent annual spending growth predicted between 2014 and 2018,[3] government is likely to make up a large proportion of this rise.

One of the historic weaknesses that the Mexican system is now having to address is that it has always been based on employment status. Most salaried or formal-sector workers are covered under one of two programmes: the Mexican Social Security Institute (IMSS) was established in 1943 for private sector, salaried and other formal workers and their families, and the Institute of Social Services and Security for Civil Servants (ISSSTE) was established in 1959 for government staff and their families. At the turn of the twenty-first century the two schemes provided cover for around 47 per cent of the population,[4] leaving half the country – the non-salaried, self-employed and unemployed – excluded from social insurance schemes. Their needs were instead covered (supposedly) by a mix of federal and state funds alongside patient fees. Essentially this meant that 50 million people were reliant on paying their own way, with many facing financial ruin.

Six Systems

Then, in 2003, under the visionary leadership of Minister of Health Julio Frenk, a new insurance scheme was launched targeting informal workers and the poor: the System for Social Protection in Health (SPSS), more commonly known as the

Seguro Popular. Premiums were means-tested, based on assets and income, and charged on a sliding scale. The stated goal of the Seguro Popular was to cover the remaining 50 million uninsured with a basic package of services by 2010. This ambitious aim was very nearly achieved: enrolee numbers reached the target in 2012 and coverage is still rising.[5] The programme places a major emphasis on preventative healthcare, including maternal and child health, and can count among its successes the elimination of the coverage gap between indigenous and non-indigenous Mexicans.[6]

Seguro Popular required major political commitment and a significant amount of new public investment. This was partly achieved by Frenk successfully making the case for healthcare as a wealth-creating industry and engine for (rather than drag on) economic growth.

As successful as the Seguro has been, it only sought to compound the divisions and fragmentations of Mexico's now six healthcare systems: The IMSS, ISSSTE, SPSS, plus separate schemes for the state oil company, armed forces and navy (known as PEMEX, SEDENA and SEMAR respectively). Each have their institutions, networks of hospitals, clinics and pharmacies, and virtually all patients are barred from using any other service. This creates huge fragmentation and waste, with an oversupply of care in some areas and a shortage in others. There are too many hospitals, too little primary care and the quality of services varies considerably.

From Coverage to Quality

When Enrique Peña Nieto successfully ran for president in 2012 he promised another round of healthcare reform to establish a truly universal system. The subsequent National Development Plan (Plan Nacional de Desarrollo 2013–18) and the Programme for the Health Sector promoted the two key ideas of convergence and portability. Convergence meaning the bringing together of Mexico's six schemes into a single universal social security system, and portability meaning patients can decide for themselves which scheme's services to seek care from.

Ending the rigid division between the schemes would greatly improve access while cutting the administration costs which currently absorb 11 per cent of spending.[7] However, it has been estimated that establishing such a scheme would cost 3 to 5 per cent of GDP, which is not currently achievable. The 'portability' element of the proposals may end up being used as an interim stage.

Frenk has argued that there are three stages to Mexico's drive for universal health coverage. The first step is universal enrolment, achieved in 2012, and the second universal coverage which he says the country is 'pretty much there' on. The third and next stage he describes as 'coverage with quality', which means a much-needed focus on improving standards across the services available. Variation is high, with differences both between schemes and between the 31 administrative regions to which many system management responsibilities are devolved. A programme of quality indicators and accreditation was introduced during the mid-2000s but there is a great deal more to do to bring provision up to a consistently acceptable standard.

Public Health Challenges

Despite commendable achievements in coverage, the well-being of Mexico's people is held back by public health threats that would challenge even the best systems. Average life expectancy has increased from 70.7 years in 1990 to 77.4 in 2015[8] but the increase has been slower than in many comparable countries, with non-communicable disease, violence and road deaths a major drag on progress.

Mexico is the world's fattest country on some measures (the highest proportion of overweight adults and the second-highest proportion of obesity), with around a third of men, women and children being obese.[9] This is creating a huge current and coming burden of diabetes and hypertension. In response, in 2013 the government launched the National Strategy for the Prevention and Control of Overweight, Obesity and Diabetes. This included health promotion campaigns and taxes on sugary soft drinks and junk food. The taxes are forecast to earn the government around US$1 billion a year[10] and early successes on the demand side have been reported, with sales of Coca Cola and other soft drinks down up to seven per cent in the first year of the policy.[11]

Another major threat is the staggering levels of violence affecting certain parts of the country. In 2010, 12.2 per cent of all deaths in Mexico were homicides, with regions such as Chihuahua reporting that 45 per cent of all deaths in men were murders.[12] The problem has spiralled out of control, with the national homicide rate doubling between 2007 and 2012, over which time 136,234 people were killed, with at least a further 30,000 missing.[13] Understandably, this is being treated as a law enforcement issue rather than a health issue but, whichever service takes the lead, the government needs to find a way of improving the security and order it can provide its citizens.

One piece of good news is that Mexico has the lowest proportion of smokers in the OECD, at less than 12 per cent.[14]

Low-cost Innovation

There are early signs that Mexico is becoming a fertile environment for innovations in health service delivery and new models of care. Both telecoms providers and retail pharmacies have begun entering the market. Walmart has partnered with local organisation Previta to offer primary care at its in-store pharmacies and there has been speculation that hospitals may seek alliances with retail chains to expand delivery networks and cut costs.[15]

Another innovation is MedicallHome, which provides a basic package of telephone-based primary healthcare advice to one million Mexican households for a monthly fee of US$5. Lines are staffed by paramedics and around two-thirds of calls are resolved on the phone. If further care is needed, MedicallHome refers them to a large network of affiliated providers, often at a discount to their usual price.[16]

One provider focusing specifically on the chronic disease challenge is a chain of low-cost diabetes clinics known as Clínicas del Azúcar.[17] Services include screening and consultations provided for an annual fee of roughly US$70–US$260. The aim is to build 50 clinics in the coming years. Clínicas del Azúcar claim that each patient who joins reduces the chances of developing a diabetes-related complication by half, while their services reduce costs by around two-thirds.

Mexico is also experimenting with the use of community health workers to support people with chronic conditions such as hypertension and diabetes.[18] These 'acompañantes' are currently based in rural and remote communities in the south. They make weekly visits to check on their patients' health and help to educate them about their condition, such as the need for exercise or a change of diet. They also liaise with doctors. Pay for the community health workers is usually in kind, such as food. They are invariably women, as it is more socially acceptable for a woman to visit a man at home than for a man to visit a woman, so the acompañantes represent a small step in improving the education and employment prospects for women. The scheme is cheap to run, makes the best of local skills and resources and does not depend on doctors and nurses, who are in short supply in the country. The programme is being driven by the non-profit Partners in Health and early successes are prompting calls for expansions to other parts of Mexico.

Finally, since 1997 Mexico has been a pioneer of large-scale conditional cash transfers as a means of combatting poverty. The Oportunidades programme sends money directly to poor families on the condition of certain behaviours such as vaccinating their children, sending them to school and ensuring they are properly fed.

Healthcare Tourism

At the other end of the healthcare spectrum, Mexico is becoming a destination for healthcare tourism. This growing trade is fuelled by Mexicans in the US, who return home because they do not have medical insurance there, and by Americans who are attracted by the prospect of high-quality care at much lower cost than in their own country: savings can be as high as 90 per cent.[19] Services being sought range from elective surgery to cosmetic and dental procedures and are often combined with more usual tourist activities. In 2011 the country came second in the Economist Intelligence Unit's ranking of medical tourism potential (after France) owing to its low costs, above-average (but unspectacular) quality and proximity to the US.[20]

Conclusion

Mexico is part way through an ambitious programme of reform to achieve universal healthcare for its people. Progress so far has been very good but the next stage – from coverage to quality, converging its six systems and overcoming immense public health challenges – is likely to be a far greater test. Imaginative use of public policy and innovations in healthcare delivery should give cause for optimism but the scale of these need to be expanded rapidly if the system is to have any chance of outrunning growing problems. Spending remains low and access continues to be a serious difficulty for poor and remote areas. Ultimately, funding truly universal healthcare will depend on growing the economy.

References

1 World Bank statistics, Total health expenditure (% of GDP) (World Bank, 2013).

2 Economist Intelligence Unit, Healthcare industry briefing: Mexico (EIU, 2014).

3 EIU, 2014.

4 Manatt Jones Global Strategies, Mexican health system: Challenges and opportunities (MJGS, 2015).

5 Pharmaboardroom, Interview with Julio Frenk, Dean – Harvard T.H. Chan School of Public Health (pharmaboardroom.com, 6 March 2015).

6 World Bank, Seguro Popular: Health coverage for all in Mexico (World Bank, 2015).

7 Economist Intelligence Unit, Healthcare industry briefing: Mexico (EIU, 2014).

8 World Bank statistics, Life expectancy at birth (World Bank, 1990 & 2013).

9 World Obesity Federation, World obesity map (WOF, 2012).

10 Martin E. & Cattan N., Mexico tackles obesity epidemic with tax on junk food (*Bloomberg Business*, 29 October 2013).

11 Guthrie A., Survey shows Mexicans drinking less soda after tax (*Wall Street Journal*, 13 October 2014).

12 Gamlin J., 'Violence and homicide in Mexico: A global health issue' in *The Lancet*, 385 (2015).

13 Human Rights Watch, Vanished: The disappeared of Mexico's drug war (HRW, 2014).

14 OECD Statistics, Tobacco consumption among adults (% daily smokers) (OECD, 2012).

15 Pharmaboardroom, Interview with José Alarcón Irigoyen, Partner & Leader of the Healthcare Practice – PwC Mexico (pharmaboardroom.com, 6 March 2015).

16 Leadbeater C., The future of healthcare: Life-saving innovations for the bottom billion (*The Guardian*, 29 September 2014).

17 Center for Health Market Innovations, Clinicas del Azucar (CHMI, 2014).

18 Partners in Health, Community Health Worker programme expands in Mexico (PIH, 2014).

19 Manatt Jones Global Strategies, Mexican health system: Challenges and opportunities (MJGS, 2015).

20 Economist Intelligence Unit, Travelling for health: The potential for medical tourism, (EIU, 2011).

26 Brazil
Order and progress?

The motto 'Ordem e Progresso' (order and progress) runs through the middle of the Brazilian flag. While Brazil's economic success has now faltered it still needs to pay close attention to the development of its health system, which has rightly been celebrated as a progressive force in developing countries but whose early successes risk being undermined.

Created by the 1988 constitution, Sistema Único de Saúde (Unified Health System, or SUS) is one of the largest public health systems in the world. It aims to provide comprehensive universal care based on the principle of health as a citizen's right and the state's duty. Health services are free at the point of use, financed through general taxation. Each level of government has to earmark a minimum portion of its revenues for health.

Primary Care Backbone

Primary care is the backbone of the SUS. The Programa Saúde da Família (Family Health Programme, or PSF) works through family health teams which usually comprise a doctor, a nurse, an auxiliary and six community health workers. They are assigned to specific families (around 1,000 per team) and provide coordinated and integrated care as well as health promotion. Within 30 years the number of family health teams has increased from 4,000 to more than 35.000.[1] They now reach 57 per cent of the 200 million population and are particularly focused on supporting poor communities in the favelas on the peripheries of cities and in the countryside.[2]

The successes of Brazil's healthcare system are numerous and substantial. Since the year 2000, infant mortality has more than halved[3] and life expectancy has increased from 69 to 74 years.[4] Equally important, disparities in health outcomes in different parts of the country and between wealthier and poorer communities have become less pronounced. SUS has played an important role in these achievements.

The quality and impact of some of Brazil's national health programmes are internationally admired, such as those for immunisation, tobacco control and AIDS, with free access to antiretroviral drugs. Brazil has one of the world's highest vaccination rates,[5] which has been key to the dramatic fall in infant and child mortality.

The rapid expansion of primary care has led to fewer people reporting difficulties in getting care, although access remains an issue, notably for diagnostic examinations and high-tech equipment.

The country's major diseases are not dissimilar to those of many developed economies, with circulatory and respiratory illnesses and cancers figuring prominently and a worrying rise in obesity, heart disease and diabetes. According to the International Diabetes Federation, 8.7 per cent of Brazil's population had diabetes in 2014, not far behind the US (9.4 per cent).[6] Brazil differs from Europe in its higher-than-average deaths from trauma and violence – road accidents and murders – and lower levels of people aged 65 and over, just 8 per cent.[7]

Civil Unrest

The problem that Brazil now faces is that it is no longer a developing country but a sizeable economic force. Its economic growth – which was 7.5 per cent in 2010 but has since slowed substantially and is expected to be almost flat in 2015 – will need to be matched by a renewed focus on healthcare just as the system shows signs of stress in its politics, funding and the way care is provided.

During the massive protests in June 2013, triggered in part by spending on the football World Cup, voters demanded improvements in the healthcare system. In recent years healthcare has routinely topped polls of voters' concerns. One of the biggest problems is a massive shortage of doctors. This is particularly felt in city slums and the remote Amazon region, where doctors are unwilling to work because of poor equipment and facilities. Medical students are reluctant to specialise in family and community medicine.

Cuban Doctors

Ministers responded quickly to the protests, introducing a programme called Mais Médicos – 'more doctors' – to hire local and foreign doctors to work in poor and remote areas. By the end of 2014 around 15,000 new doctors, more than three-quarters of them from Cuba, had been enrolled.[8] Others came from Argentina, Portugal and Spain. In January 2015 the government announced a new wave of overseas doctor employment, again aimed at deprived areas.

The overseas recruitment drive met determined opposition from Brazilian medical organisations. The relatively low pay and restrictions on where the overseas doctors could work prompted overblown comparisons with slave labour. The doctors' associations do not hesitate to use their political influence; in the past their lobbying has undermined nurses' training and secured a ban on anyone who was not a doctor prescribing a drug.

The government has also announced new medical schools to train thousands of additional doctors and training is being extended from six to eight years to include two years working in public service posts. This could add 36,000 working students to the system by 2021. A government minister said the compulsory training in public hospitals was inspired by the NHS. Opponents claim potential students will be put off by the length of training.

Big disparities in provision persist. Cities such as São Paulo, for example, have plenty of hospitals, although public hospitals in major cities frequently suffer from overcrowding and there can be long delays for surgery. But in backwater states in the Amazon, even ill-equipped clinics are scarce.

There is evidence of weaknesses in medical training and quality assurance, with ministers having argued that the priority is providing enough doctors to ensure medical cover in rural areas. In 2011 the Ministry of Health launched the Health Care Network Training and Quality Improvement Programme, the QualiSUS-Rede, but there is a long way to go in developing robust quality and safety systems. Too few clinics or hospitals are engaged in developing such systems and connections between research, teaching and practice are weak. Failures in hospital management also need to be addressed, including financial and administrative systems and training.

Total spending on healthcare in 2012 was around 9.7 per cent of GDP, higher than the Latin American average.[9] The Economist Intelligence Unit estimates that spending in Brazil will rise to US$233 billion or 3 per cent per year to 2019, compared with economic growth of around 2 per cent, implying funding problems ahead.[10]

With the difficulties SUS is experiencing, it is not surprising that 24 per cent of the population has private health insurance,[11] with numerous private hospitals competing for customers. Many members of the growing middle class regard health insurance as a mark of their prosperity. Private healthcare has grown to the extent that government now only accounts for about 48 per cent of national healthcare spending;[12] the OECD average is 70 per cent.

Given the funding pressures and the growth in private healthcare, a way forward would be for the public healthcare system to form partnerships with the private sector. Many parts of Brazil are experimenting with public–private partnerships to build and run facilities, although the public sector has a lot to learn about managing these relationships and contracts.

Back to the Twentieth Century?

Perhaps the greatest risk to Brazil's healthcare system is that the growing dominance of the acute sector threatens to take its progressive models of care backwards to a twentieth-century model based around unaffordable hospitals. To counter this, a new vision needs to be fashioned for the country's healthcare development over the next decade.

In October 2014 President Dilma Rousseff, whose Workers' Party had already been in power for 12 years, was narrowly re-elected. She has promised further expansion of community health but her most urgent priority is to rekindle economic growth. While much of the political debate has been focused on fiscal policy and currency issues, difficulties in sustaining healthcare investment could expose some of the underlying fragility of the health system. This, in turn, risks limiting long-run economic performance. SUS – a great national healthcare innovation a quarter of a century ago – needs to refresh its vision. It needs to maintain its strong focus on primary care and prevention while continuing to improve access and addressing shortfalls in staffing, training, quality and management.

What does this mean in practice? Some argue that the improvement of the Brazilian healthcare system is just a matter of government will and more spending. I'm not sure it is as straightforward as that; we should be cautious of offering too much advice from a traditional European perspective. Better family and community health medicine and a more 'activist' payer approach with the independent sector should be central priorities for federal and state health agencies.

Redefining the relationship with the private sector will be key to the next stage of development. Instinctive suspicion of private healthcare needs to give way to a more collaborative and transparent relationship; the private healthcare market is now too big to be seen simply as a parallel system. This will require vision and political will. Yet, attitudes are beginning to soften; in January 2015 a law was passed relaxing restrictions on foreign investment in healthcare, including hospitals, clinics and research. This is seen by the government as a way of facilitating technology and skills transfer into the health system as well as raising further financing.[13]

Equally, the rise and consolidation of the private health insurance market should be subject to regulation that stimulates the design of a higher-value, lower-cost model of care that looks less to the economically inefficient hospital and fee-per-service system, developed in the US throughout the twentieth century, and more to a future reflecting the culture and character of the new economic powerhouses known as the BRICS. Following the old US model would drive costs and care design in the wrong direction.

Conclusion

Brazil is moving from being a developing country to a major world economy with a healthcare system that can claim a number of successes. It has impressive prevention through vaccination programmes and tobacco control and has built strong foundations in primary care. While the economy was buoyant it made considerable strides towards its goal of universal provision free at the point of need but access and quality in the city favelas and remote regions of this vast country are still inadequate. Now that the economy has slowed, the development of healthcare has lost momentum and Brazil needs renewed political vision to pick up progress.

Nonetheless, developed countries would do well to learn from some of the best characteristics of Brazilian healthcare, particularly the principles of the extended clinical teams delivering the family health programme and the resolute focus on large-scale preventative and public health campaigns.

References

1 Gragnolati et al., Twenty years of health system reform in Brazil (World Bank, 2013) p. 2.

2 Araujo et al., Contracting for primary care in Brazil: The cases of Bahia and Rio de Janeiro (World Bank, 2014).

3 World Bank statistics, Infant mortality rate (per live 1000 births) (World Bank, 2013).

4 Economic Intelligence Unit data (January 2015).

5 World Bank statistics, Immunization: Measles (% of children ages 12–23 months) (World Bank, 2013).

6 International Diabetes Federation, IDF Diabetes Atlas: 6th edition (IDF, 2014).

7 World Bank statistics, Population aged 65 and above (% of total) (World Bank, 2013).

8 Whitney W.T., Cuban doctors attend to Brazil's underserved (People's World, 28 March 2014).

9 World Bank statistics, Total health expenditure (% of GDP) (World Bank, 2013).

10 Economic Intelligence Unit data (EIU, January 2015).

11 Economist Intelligence Unit, Healthcare briefing: Brazil (EIU, October 2014).

12 World Bank statistics, Health expenditure: Public (% of total health expenditure) (World Bank, 2013).

13 KPMG Brazil, Brazilian healthcare: Regulatory change results in investment opportunities for foreign organizations (KPMG, 2015).

Global Challenges

27 Universal Healthcare

Triumph of political will

I have walked through the shanty towns of India, townships of South Africa and favelas of Brazil and have marvelled at the marbled corridors of private hospitals in the same countries, wondering how these groups of people and societies co-exist. It is a deeply disturbing and provoking experience and has certainly made me a passionate advocate for universal healthcare. The potential for social instability from these inequalities in care is high, a fact not lost on the political classes crossing all continents from Brazil, Mexico and Chile to South Africa, Rwanda and Ghana, Turkey and Saudi Arabia through to India, China, Indonesia and Thailand to name but a few. It has been estimated by a recent Chatham House report that the minimum public expenditure required to provide an adequate package of health services for a country's entire population would be US$86 per person per year.[1] While some countries have achieved miracles for less, politicians are starting to realise that investment in healthcare for all is a value and not just a cost.

Many commentators and policy-makers now believe that universal healthcare is an idea whose time has finally come. From the World Bank to the United Nations through to WHO, people can rightly point to the moral, social, economic and political benefits of the concept, which WHO defines as 'access to key promotive, preventive, curative and rehabilitative health interventions for all at an affordable cost, thereby achieving equity in access'. The Director-General of WHO has gone on record to say that universal healthcare 'is the single, most powerful concept that public health has to offer',[2] while the President of the World Bank, Jim Yong Kim, recently declared in the *Financial Times* that 'the economic case for universal health coverage is strong'.[3] The pivotal position of universal healthcare in the Sustainable Development Goals will further secure its place at the heart of the global development agenda for the next decade and beyond.

It has been estimated that approximately 40 per cent of the world's countries have universal healthcare[4] but these levels are set to expand because of two forces which are, paradoxically, diametrically opposed. First, the growth of capitalism and globalisation has resulted in unprecedented levels of wealth and a rapidly expanding middle class which is demanding more from governments and consuming more from services. Roughly, just over a billion people

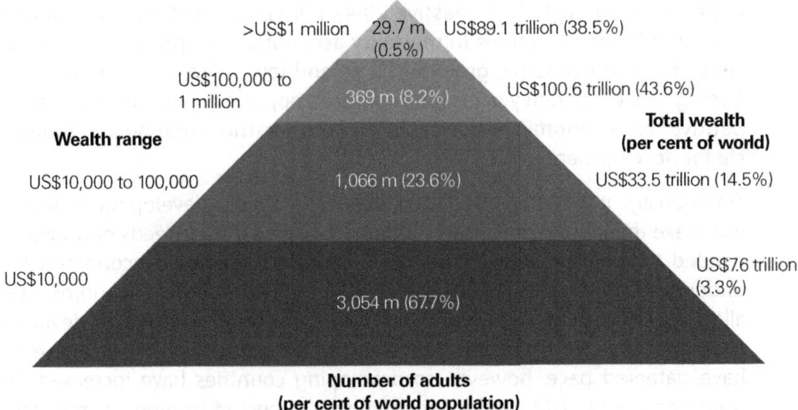

Figure 26.1 The global wealth pyramid

now have annual earnings between US$10,000 and US$100,000 which places them within the middle-class bracket. However, nearly 70 per cent of the world's population still exists on less than US$10,000 per year, one billion people lack access to basic healthcare and 100 million are impoverished every year through catastrophic financial hardship associated with healthcare costs.[5] These two forces – globalisation and wealth inequality – will create fertile ground for the development of universal healthcare but its successful introduction cannot be taken for granted. Above all else, the presence or absence of political will and vision will determine whether citizens of the planet will enjoy a fundamental human necessity. We still live in a world where the average life expectancy between rich and poor countries can differ by as much as 40 years, a terrible waste of potentially productive human capacity and capability.[6]

Health Spending is a Value, Not a Cost

The arguments for universal healthcare are overwhelming. The excellent Lancet Commission on Investing for Health makes the case most persuasively, outlining the ways in which health gain has a direct impact on a country's GDP.[7] These are: productivity (people enjoying decent health are more productive and take less sick leave); education (healthier children turn up for school and learn skills); investment (people think about the future more, spend less on 'catastrophic' health costs and save when they look forward to longer life); and demographics (healthy life improves the ratio of work to dependency). It has been estimated that a one-year increase in life expectancy can increase GDP per capita by 4 per cent, while improved health in the workforce can improve productivity by a massive 20-47 per cent.[8] The Lancet Commission also noted that reductions in mortality accounted for approximately 11 per cent of recent economic growth in low- and low–middle-income countries. Average life expectancy gains for a country's population will enhance its competitiveness, economic performance and output, thus creating a virtuous circle for development.

Traditionally, it has been assumed that only rapidly developing economies will make the leap to universal healthcare because the proceeds of growth are needed to fund expanded coverage. Historically, emerging economies have underinvested in health. In 2012, according to BCG, emerging economies' GDP allocation for health was around 5.6 per cent, around half that of developed countries.[9] As the arguments about health investment and wealth creation have gathered pace, however, so developing countries have increased their spending. Up to 2022, health expenditure is expected to grow even faster, at 10.7 per cent compared with 3.7 per cent in developed economies for the same period. In 2022, global health spend is projected to pass US$12 trillion, of which 30 per cent will be committed by emerging countries.

Donor funding for health has also increased dramatically as the relationship of health and wealth has become better understood. Overseas aid for health quadrupled between 2002 and 2010, with the emergence of new global health funding streams of an unprecedented size, such as the United States President's Emergency Plan for AIDS Relief (PEPFAR) and the Global Fund to Fight AIDS, Tuberculosis and Malaria. Growth of these programmes has stalled since the global financial crisis but, alongside economic infrastructure projects, health remains an almost uniquely favoured area of investment for international donors.

The Need for Political Will

Confidence in global growth will help developing nations make the case for health investment but political vision will determine its trajectory. In every single case where universal healthcare has been advanced, the leadership, will and vision of politicians has been essential, along with promising economic circumstances. While there are other ingredients that will ensure good implementation and execution, only the political process can determine how a country decides to prioritise resources. Bismarck was the first politician to pioneer universal social insurance, in the late nineteenth century, and this was followed by various waves of political action after the Second World War starting with Attlee and Bevan in the UK in 1948 and moving through the decades: for example, Sweden and Chile in the 1950s, Japan and Denmark in the 1960s, South Korea and Italy in the 1970s, Spain and Australia in the 1980s, Israel and Taiwan in the 1990s, and more recently Thailand in 2000, China in 2009, the US in 2012 and Indonesia in 2014.

In a paper presented at the World Innovation Summit for Health 2015 by Sir David Nicholson and Lord Ara Darzi, the authors note the critical role of political will because the transition towards universal health is an intensely political act, redistributing both health benefits and financial burdens.[10] It has been opposed by many powerful groups, including some doctors' groups in countries such as South Africa, Brazil, Nigeria and China.

Central to political will and direction in developing countries is the emerging middle class. This group more than any other holds the balance of power in the development of universal healthcare, as their newfound economic, political and social power can be used as a force either for conservatism or progress. In countries where the middle class have sought to purchase insurance or self-pay for care in times of sickness, efforts to establish universal healthcare have often been thwarted as there is less incentive to extend coverage to other segments of the population. I have seen how pernicious this can be in countries such as India, Brazil and Nigeria, where the latter only has 5 per cent coverage despite proclamations that it is seeking to adopt universal healthcare. However, in Rwanda coverage has exceeded 90 per cent because a more robust approach made insurance membership mandatory with heavily subsidised premiums.

Breadth Before Depth

Experience around the world shows that one of the keys to winning over a critical mass of popular and political support for universal healthcare is to aim for breadth first and depth later. Some countries have attempted to develop a fully comprehensive package of care for particular sections of their population, but more often than not these have run into the ground as implementation is overwhelmingly complex and public optimism turns to frustration during the long wait. Far better to take a 'shallow-base' approach – provide a small number of benefits to all citizens quickly, build support from a strong community and primary care base, and create a virtuous cycle of popular encouragement and increasing political confidence. This is one of the keys to China's successful journey so far: giving a basic level of coverage to all, then developing its depth.

It is at this point that politicians, policy-makers and practitioners have difficult choices to make regarding the supply and provision of healthcare. There is an ongoing debate among low- and middle-income countries – as there is in the West – about the extent to which governments should be providers of healthcare or merely funders. While these discussions can quickly become quite ideological from both the right and left, it is my observation that achieving universal healthcare for most countries will require much greater public–private collaboration. That said, if a breadth-first approach is taken then the majority of investment for at least the first decade or so will be in improving primary and community-based care, which largely means public provision.

Whatever approach is chosen, governments will want to pay very close attention to, and in some cases control, which models of care develop. A growing number of examples around the world show how developing economies have a huge opportunity to leapfrog Western health systems, as a result of fewer impediments (less infrastructure, weaker vested interests, lower public expectations), the rapid spread of technology and the strength of 'people power'.

The graph below illustrates what is at stake and the importance of low- and middle-income countries developing lean innovative care models, rather than replicating the models (and mistakes) of the high-income countries.[11]

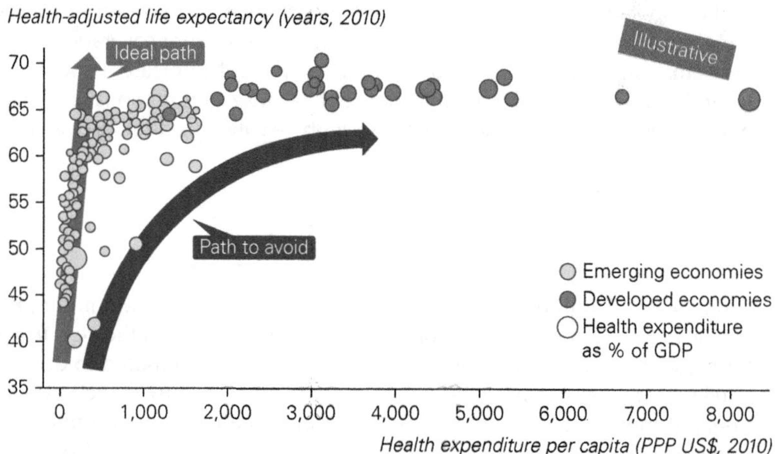

In many developing countries the instinct to replicate and imitate the health systems of the developed economies is strong but new entrants are challenging twentieth-century thinking and introducing frugal innovation which meets local needs. In many cases, high-income health systems have much to learn from these innovations in their pursuit of high-quality care at low cost.

KPMG recently convened a conference in Africa where over 50 public and private sector health leaders from across the continent discussed the provision of low-cost, high-quality healthcare. It also invited leaders from India to present their experiences of innovation, and subsequently published a report entitled *Necessity: the Mother of Innovation*.[12]

Delegates pointed to a number of areas they expected to see emerge as key features of low-cost, high-quality healthcare systems (see box).

Key aspects of 'frugal innovation', according to African healthcare leaders

- Asset-light and fit-for-use facilities and IT (not over-specified)
- Flexible, multi-tasking, team-based working
- Primary and community care
- Carer or supported services delivered in conjunction with patients
- Centralised specialist work delivered through a coordinated network of providers
- Centralisation of clinical diagnostics and support services and lean supply chains
- Strong professional management
- Communities as carers
- Education and health promotion for women

Many of these issues are also of critical importance to advanced economies but the scale, scope and speed of change in developing countries can be impressive. Many existing models are clear and disciplined about the range of services they offer or the population and disease segment they serve. In these cases, streamlining and standardising patient flows are crucial.

For example, Glocal Healthcare in India was founded in 2010 and established standardised diagnosis and management protocols for the 42 diseases from which 95 per cent of the population suffered.[13] This enabled low-cost or leased facilities to be created, service and consumables costs to be reduced, traditional workflow patterns to be modified, and skills to be maximised for nurse practitioners and physician assistants alike. Glocal has adopted a standardised Medical Diagnosis & Management System that is connected to the Hospital Management Information System. This is an artificial intelligence system that helps with diagnosis, choosing medication and preventing adverse drug interactions. While doctors still exercise their judgement, this makes the entire process of diagnosis and management fully transparent and documented. It ensures that an accurate diagnosis is quickly determined without unnecessary medicines, laboratory tests and procedures, thus further streamlining healthcare delivery and its costs. There are many similar examples of standardisation and process streamlining, such as Narayana, Aravind Eye Care and Apollo (see Chapter 9: India).

While many models are looking for the lowest costs per episode or transaction, some emerging strategies in India and Africa are focused on improving value across the continuum of care, including greater population health management. I have seen two approaches which offer great promise and certainly move away from acute or tertiary-dominated systems. The first model is being tested in India and looks at the development of mobile phone-linked insurance and health delivery. In this model the individual pays a monthly fee or per-use charge and receives advice from health professionals in call centres. This call centre works to protocols covering the main conditions and ailments and is directed by a small group of doctors who support a wider group of other clinicians and clerical staff. The call centres have a strong distribution channel to pharmacies. Patients in effect by-pass primary care and hospitals to obtain their diagnosis, advice and medications from local pharmacies when telephone calls are insufficient. This approach has also been successful in places such as Mexico where disease-specific care givers provide advice and treatment via the telephone and through strong distribution channels. Costs are dramatically lower and consumer satisfaction is high.

The second model, which often builds on the first approach, looks at covering a population or network. For example, Vaatsalya Healthcare was founded in 2005 and set up to provide accessible, affordable and efficient care to the rural and semi-urban people of India living in Tier II and Tier III cities (those behind the big six such as Delhi and Mumbai).[14] Vaatsalya says that 'while 70 per cent of India is living in semi-urban and rural areas, 80 per cent of India's healthcare facilities are located in urban or metro areas'. They provide a service that is subsidised by the wealthier parts of the community and aimed at the lower-middle class and those below the poverty line. They have developed an integrated system of community-based services backed up by a network of primary care clinics which, in turn, are linked to ambulatory care facilities and hospitals. They seek to provide as much advice and care in the community as possible. The big advantage for patients is markedly reduced travel time and costs and a corresponding reduction in lost wages incurred through time off work. Some global private equity players are now developing similar models and are looking to trial these systems across the major urban areas in developing countries.

No Health Without a Workforce

Finally, any country that wishes to develop universal healthcare will confront the problem of skill and workforce shortages. There is a saying that 'there is no health without a workforce' and it is well recognised that even in countries that are able to finance universal health coverage there may not be the health workers available to deliver it. For example, sub-Saharan Africa has approximately 25 per cent of the world's disease burden but only 3 per cent of the health workforce.[15] Conversely, countries such as the US and UK attract skilled health workers from across the world, often from developing countries facing far greater shortages. It is now estimated that one in four or one in five doctors in the US and UK comes from abroad. Globalisation, urbanisation and the increasing cross-national transfer of technology, expertise and patients will further compound these pressures. WHO estimated that there is a global shortage of approximately 7.2 million health workers, rising to 13 million by 2035, which represents a 15 per cent shortage worldwide.[16] If the US cannot find enough doctors, what chance do developing countries have?

The answer is to do something different. Lord Nigel Crisp's seminal publication *Turning the World Upside Down* points to the many examples of innovative 'task sharing' in low- and middle-income countries.[17] He describes how low-skilled workers are being trained to perform common procedures with quality and efficiency, while the all-too-rare doctors focus on the area requiring their breadth of expertise. Patients and communities themselves are also being seen as a vital part of the healthcare workforce.

Conclusion

Universal healthcare is an idea whose time has come. With funding for health growing and rising public expectations driving up political ambitions, my hope is that we will see hundreds of millions more people gain access to healthcare over the coming decade. A great many barriers stand in the way, but many more examples show how these can be overcome. What is clear is that healthcare for the next billion of the world's people will look very different to the healthcare most people currently see. It will be shaped as much by telecommunications companies and communities themselves as ministries of health and large hospitals. It will depend on new models of care that even countries that have enjoyed universal coverage for decades have much to learn from: standardising processes, innovating environments, streamlining procurement, and using technology to drive efficiency in order to empower the workforce and mobilise communities.

References

1 McIntyre D. and Meheus F., Fiscal space for domestic funding of health and other social services (Chatham House, 2014).

2 World Health Organization, Ministerial meeting on universal health coverage: Opening remarks of the Director-General (WHO, 2013).

3 Kim J.Y., There is a strong economic case for universal health coverage (*Financial Times*, 16 October 2014).

4 McKee M. et al., 'Universal health coverage: A quest for all countries but under threat in some' in *Value in Health*, (16) S39–S45 (2013).

5 World Health Organization. The World Health Report: Health systems financing: The path to universal coverage (WHO, 2010).

6 Shorrocks A., Davies J.B. and Lluberas R., The global wealth report 2014 (Credit Suisse AG, 2014).

7 Jamison D.T. et al., 'Global health 2035: a world converging within a generation' in *The Lancet*, 382 (9908) pp. 1898–1955.

8 Bloom D. et al., 'The effect of health on economic growth: A production function approach' in *World Development*, 32 (1) 1–13 (2004).

9 World Economic Forum and Boston Consulting Group, Health systems leapfrogging in emerging economies (WEF, 2014).

[10] Nicholson D. et al., Delivering universal health coverage: A guide for policy makers (WISH, 2015).

[11] WEF (2014) p. 6.

[12] KPMG International, Necessity: The mother of innovation (KPMG, 2014).

[13] Ibid., p. 35.

[14] Ibid., p. 40

[15] Crisp N. and Chen L., 'Global supply of health professionals' in *New England Journal of Medicine*, 370 (10) 2014.

[16] World Health Organization, A universal truth: No health without a workforce (WHO, 2013).

[17] Crisp N., *Turning the world upside down: The search for global health in the 21st century* (CRC Press: London, 2010).

28 Same Problem, Different Country

The paradox of change

In a world confronted by war, political instability, economic insecurity, climate change, globalisation and the threat of terror, it is to the credit of the World Economic Forum that it dedicated some of its time to look at the important as well as urgent and politically pressing matters that confront global leaders today. Health and well-being is one of the most important aspects of any country and it is frequently cited as one of the top three most pressing concerns for citizens. In this light, it is not surprising that its importance is rising within the political class as well as healthcare professionals and the population at large. It is, however, more than a little odd that countries have not collaborated to a much higher degree to seek sustainable healthcare solutions and implement them. Innovation and adoption are two sides of the same sustainable healthcare coin.

In its report *The Great Transformation: Shaping New Models*, the World Economic Forum brought together the issues of the growing financial burden of health systems from ageing, lifestyles and public expectations and the need to develop a more sustainable way of managing them. It concluded: 'The magnitude of health financing challenges suggest that incremental solutions may not be enough; however, a shared vision of new models for health systems does not yet exist'.[1]

More global research, development and collaboration is needed on business and care model innovation in health. I am a member of the World Economic Forum Global Agenda Council on the Future of the Health Sector. Fifteen health experts from around the world gather to consider why sustainable change in healthcare is slow, fragmented and difficult to achieve. We have identified that a lack of alignment between payers, providers, patients, professionals, policymakers, politicians, the public and the press is a serious drag on innovation and progress. In my opening chapter 'The Perfect Health System', I explained that no country can boast perfection but argued that many countries can illustrate brilliant examples of great healthcare. All these local health system successes were designed, built, implemented and sustained by human beings overcoming multiple challenges. Imagine the enormous potential for good if these local examples can be harnessed and introduced at scale for the wider benefit of population health.

This question has continually exercised me during the past six years. What continues to strike me is that organisations have a strong sense of their own value and an unswerving commitment to high-quality care but little appreciation of the worth and the true strategic value of others in the local, regional or national health systems of which they are but one important part. I have often been struck by the way companies operating in industries as diverse as telecommunications, transport and defence manage to collaborate in a competitive environment, yet health organisations find collaboration immensely difficult even when they are not competing.

This fragmentation, at both a policy and practice level, not only hampers high-quality, universal healthcare but also wastes scarce resources and frequently results in higher costs to patients, the wider public and taxpayers alike. The antidote to fragmentation is integration and this is, arguably, the most hotly discussed and fashionable concept in healthcare today.

Four Ingredients of High-quality Systems

In its landmark report *Crossing the Quality Chasm* the highly respected Institute of Medicine in America identified four vital ingredients for high-quality systems and care.[2]

The first vital ingredient is vision – more specifically, what has subsequently been called the 'triple aim' of better experience of care (safe, effective, patient-centred, timely, efficient and equitable), better health for the population and lower per capita costs. The paper notes that reforms which only pay superficial concern to these high-level aims often fail in their sustainability.

Second, focus on the design of the clinical care process from the patient's perspective. Clinical microsystems, the Institute of Medicine argues, are famously unstable, unreliable and highly variable in cost and safety. Clinicians have a duty of care to actively participate in quality improvement initiatives in order to lead.

Third, care organisations need to be linked and integrated into care systems. As Don Berwick and others have argued in the *New England Journal of Medicine*, 'we need organisations large enough to be accountable for the full continuum of care as well as for achieving the triple aim'.[3] They believe that high-performing health systems will only be established if 'integrated delivery systems become the mainstay of organisational design'.

The Institute of Medicine's fourth ingredient is the wider environment which includes regulation, education, legal and financial systems. They make the obvious but difficult point that wider environmental forces need to be aligned and facilitate collaboration and cooperation among healthcare professionals and across healthcare organisations.

Every country's health system is a product of its cultural, social, economic and political circumstances but often their high-level policy goals are similar: improved access to health services; improved quality and efficiency; and greater patient and consumer choice or control over services – all potently mixed with money and political and professional power. There are ten elements that I have repeatedly come across which helped deliver the four ingredients of high-quality, affordable healthcare:

Similar solutions, different countries

1. Strong health promotion and illness prevention and good joined-up well-being policies and plans across the public and private sector.
2. Excellent population and patient segmentation and stratification techniques to encourage and support citizens and patients to live actively, all supported by the latest technology.
3. A scaled-up primary care system with access to speedy diagnostics and therapeutics provided in suitable facilities and supported through integrated community and pharmacy health teams.
4. Simultaneously localised and centralised clinical services which put care in communities where possible but concentrate care where clinically necessary to improve patient outcomes and efficiency.
5. Excellent care plans and pathways developed by clinicians and supported by improvement science, and which are accountable and transparent.
6. Workforce motivation and development that looks at the sensible delegation and demarcation of skills from the patient's perspective and not just the producer's.
7. Strong tertiary centres that act as health systems, linking secondary and primary care services and facilitated by leading-edge paramedic services that provide care on the spot.
8. Integrated health and aged care provided seamlessly from the home and funded fairly through adequate financing from public and private sources, as necessary.
9. Community-based mental health services which recognise the personal and economic importance of mental health.
10. Above all else, a health system which treats patients as active partners in their care (and communities as carers), and allows individuals and carers control over their life and, ultimately, their death.

The Barriers to High-Quality Care

What stops other well-educated, highly skilled and supremely well-motivated people in teams making health and care higher quality, better integrated, less fragmented and ultimately more sustainable? Ironically, the short answer is the organisations in which they work and the pressures, incentives and regulatory circumstances in which they operate.

In essence, there are three compounding problems which inhibit large-scale, sustainable change. First, organisational myopia. Organisations have a tendency to think they are basically good but the health system in which they operate is poor at supporting their success.

Second, the ability for transactional reform to trump transformational change. I define transaction as 'doing things better' and transformation as 'doing better things'. Often, it is easier and less threatening to make seemingly important but small changes than it is to hold individuals, organisations or systems to account for transformational change which will produce better health, better care and better value.

Third, large-scale change is as much an emotional issue as a technical one but this is rarely prioritised. A compelling vision of a better future needs to be communicated in a way that creates energy and sustains motivation. This means that staff have to be able to relate to it, shape it and feel empowered through distributed leadership to challenge the status quo. Processes, procedures and structures need to be subordinated to, and support, the changes required and staff need to be trained, coached and held to account for progress. Simple to say, difficult to do.

It may be of some comfort to know that health is not the only industry which is stubborn to change. A recent KPMG global survey of 3,000 leading executives across 20 industries spread across the world found that board leaders were twice as likely to focus on short-term cost efficiencies in their respective organisations than they were to prepare their own organisations for major business model change. Unfortunately, when we looked at the statistics for health and life science leaders globally, we found that they were nearly three times as likely to focus on the urgent issues of today and not the important ones of tomorrow. Respondents cited the pressures and challenges of short-term politics as the principal reason for this focus. Politicians can make or break health systems but they should rarely get involved in the detailed day-to-day management.

In further global research, we asked health leaders what the principal pre-occupation of their time was and found that 85 per cent of effort was directed towards heavily operational matters such as cost reduction, income maximisation, internal quality improvement methodologies and health IT investment. Of course, some of these activities would almost certainly lend themselves to more transformational approaches but the balance of effort was primarily transactional.

Paradoxically, as the table below shows, executives frequently see the need for system-wide change before they see the need to transform their own organisations.[4]

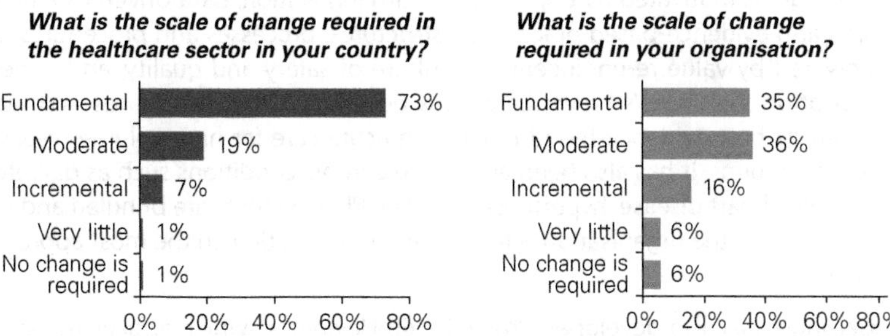

Essentially health practitioners realise the scale and size of change and transformation required but believe this is somebody else's problem. The locus for change has neither been internalised nor socialised and the inability to get groups of senior health leaders together from different sectors (purchaser, primary care, community care, hospital care or patients groups and professional regulators) to imagine what sustainable change looks like thwarts any serious attempt to transform care. When the belief that change starts with someone else is coupled with a deeply transactional mindset and culture, the force to preserve the status quo is very strong.

When we asked global leaders what could potentially align organisation and health system interests to provide better health, better care and better value the overwhelming answer was integration; 90 per cent of respondents believed integration will improve outcomes while 75 per cent thought costs would also reduce. Further, 82 per cent of participants across 30 countries believed their health system would become more integrated over the next five years. Health leaders, clinicians and managers know that integration makes strategic sense but don't know how to implement sustainable solutions when effort and focus is so short term.

Geisinger – Revealing the Paradox

There are many health systems that demonstrate excellent progress in parts of the integration journey including examples in Japan, Singapore, Spain, New Zealand and the UK, but the best system I have engaged with is Geisinger in Pennsylvania, America. It is an uplifting case study of nearly all of the elements described above and has produced great results for improved health, care and value. Founded in 1915, the Geisinger Health System provides a complete continuum of care for more than 2.6 million people. It has been listed in the 'Best

Hospitals in America' and the 'Best Doctors in America'.[5] It runs both hospitals and nursing homes, has its own health insurance plan and a physician practice group which includes primary and secondary care clinicians.

Geisinger is motivated by population health innovation, data-driven care redesign and evidence-based practice. Its structures, processes and procedures are powered by value re-engineering, a culture of safety and quality, and patient activation. Geisinger's ProvenCare® was developed from careful research and supports best evidence-based practice in acute care for high-volume disease-related groups. It has also been applied to chronic conditions such as diabetes, coronary heart disease, hypertension and COPD. Payments are bundled and the incentive for the organisation is to get care right first time in the most appropriate setting.

Geisinger has also developed ProvenHealthNavigator® which applies the same principles to primary and home care. It has a well-developed clinical information system and medical records are shared between practitioners and patients. Geisinger had the audacity to try to change the way healthcare is provided and paid for in America and it has reduced its costs and made substantial improvement to care quality and in-hospital mortality. It deserves recognition.

It has a 100-year history of providing high-quality care to the people of Pennsylvania. However, its journey to become one of the world's most innovative health systems has in large part taken place during the 15-year tenure of Glenn Steele. Speaking to Glenn about his leadership style and the lessons he has learned as President and Chief Executive from 2000 to 2015, several things stand out.

First is the remarkable staying power of him and his organisation. Glenn is only the fifth leader Geisinger has had since its establishment in 1915, and his strategy has remained remarkably consistent throughout his decade and a half at the top. The first clinical specialities to adopt ProvenCare® started in 2003 and the organisation has been working through the rest for the past 12 years – they are currently at 20. This consistency, twinned with early successes, provides an invaluable momentum that makes wider change irresistible. It also allows a powerful evidence base to be built up over time. Glenn freely admits some of the founding principles of the transformations he drove were built more on 'religious' beliefs about what better care looked like rather than hard evidence. With several years of data amassed demonstrating the value of these beliefs, however, bigger and bolder transformations could be driven through.

Making these changes required an awful lot of skill, will and time. This is the paradox of change: it requires continuity.

A second theme is the importance of periods of crisis or poor performance to Geisinger's improvement and expansion. When Glenn joined the organisation in 2000 it had recently gone through a highly problematic merger and was making 5 per cent losses across all areas of its business, necessitating workforce reductions of over 10 per cent. Curiously, it was this crisis that attracted Glenn to the position, as he saw it as an opportunity for fundamental transformation of a health system not possible in comfortable, well-established institutions. Since then, challenging performance has been a key driver of Geisinger's expansion into a number of its now 55 community sites and multiple hub hospitals. Where others might see a challenged provider, it sees a potential partner willing to transform their ways of working using the Geisinger model.

Glenn grasps the central importance of culture. He sees the rewriting of Geisinger's social contract with its employees as the foundation on which subsequent improvements were made. During the early years of change he held around 60 staff group meetings per year, to keep in touch with how change was progressing on the ground and to regularly reiterate the principles and purpose behind the new ways of working. His philosophy of innovation, intolerance of unjustified variation and not rewarding failure was not universally popular at the start but he persevered and built an integrated system which many considered to be the genesis of accountable care in America.

Conclusion

Healthcare leaders do not spend sufficient time or effort strategically imagining the future with other parts of the health system and do not place great faith in their own ability to develop and implement sustainable solutions to problems they know exist. When coupled with an inevitable desire to survive and succeed in a fairly narrow and operational set of performance metrics, it is easy to see why energy is focused on doing things better rather than doing better things. Nobody gets held to account for producing a more sustainable health system; they usually just get rewarded for surviving or thriving in the existing one.

Health leaders need to recognise that they are not alone in grappling with their health system and should not be afraid of attempting to change it, because no one has got it absolutely right. They must also recognise that the paradox of change is continuity.

References

1 World Economic Forum, The great transformation: Shaping new care models (WEF, 2011).

2 Institute of Medicine, Crossing the quality chasm: A new health system for the 21st century (IOM, 2001).

3 Fisher E.S. et al., 'Achieving health care reform: How physicians can help,' *New England Journal of Medicine*, 260, 2495–7 (2009).

4 KPMG International global crowdsourcing research, conducted June 2014.

5 *US News*, US News Best Hospitals 2014–15 (*US News*, 2014).

29 Clinical Quality
The more I know, the less I sleep

'The more I know, the less I sleep.' This great quote, from former colleague Dr David Rosser, Executive Medical Director of University Hospitals Birmingham in the UK, reflects the mix of anxiety, curiosity and drive which is an inextricable part of the quest to provide great care.

Vastly more people die each year through mistakes in their medical care than die in planes, trains and automobiles put together. For example, a review in the *Journal of Patient Safety* in 2013 estimated that more than 400,000 patients die prematurely each year in the US alone as a result of preventable harm to patients.[1] In the UK the government has estimated there are 12,000 avoidable patient deaths a year,[2] compared to road deaths of 1,700 per year.[3]

We would not fly if the current random quality controls in healthcare were adopted by the aviation industry. The humble family car is built to more exacting quality standards than most clinical systems. The essential elements of improvement – a devotion to quality, accountability, standardised processes and measurement – were adopted in other industries decades ago. They now need to be applied in healthcare systematically, with accurately reported outcomes providing the glue to bind together patients, professionals, providers and those paying for and regulating care.

It is odd that something so important and personal as healthcare does not have widely acknowledged or adopted industry standards of inspection, reporting and improvement. The troubles at the Bristol and Mid Staffordshire hospitals in the UK, the Walter Reed Army Medical Center neglect scandal in the US, and the Garling inquiry into New South Wales Public Hospitals in Australia demonstrate what can happen when outcomes are not measured, reported and analysed effectively. The tragedy of these cases is compounded by the fact that an organisational culture of denial and lack of attentiveness to patient welfare meant the concerns of staff and patients were ignored – although the very fact that we have heard of such scandals is a credit to the degree of transparency in the wider systems of these countries.

Excellence is being pursued in systems beset by an old-fashioned, individualised, craft-based culture which does not reflect what we know works better in the twenty-first century: clinical teams executing safety and improvement science on an industrial scale. In the search for an easy remedy for poor care we are distracted by ever more detailed regulations which give comfort to politicians and officials but fail to secure high quality in a sustainable fashion.

If a hospital board is to be 'in control' of quality there needs to be a culture devoted to it, staff who feel responsible and accountable, standardised and optimised processes, and systematic real-time measurement. Few, if any, of the world's healthcare leaders would claim their organisations are fully 'in control'. Even those widely acknowledged as shining examples of best practice admit they have some way to go in understanding what drives outcomes and how to measure quality and avoid harming patients. Mike Harper, Executive Dean of Clinical Practice of the US-based Mayo Clinic, explains: 'Compared to the average, we're doing pretty well; we score on the top of most lists. But are we "in control" yet? No. Are we where we want to be? No. But we're on our way. We score very high on all of these measures, yet we can do better.'

Becoming a High-reliability Provider

In a high-risk environment such as healthcare (and, indeed, in aviation, chemical processing and nuclear power), the aim is to become a 'high-reliability' provider that is focused on consistently excellent outcomes along with preventing failure. Such organisations align their leadership, core processes and measurement systems, with clear lines of accountability and a common mindset from the ground floor to the boardroom. A study of healthcare providers by KPMG showed four phases that they progress through to reaching a status of high reliability:[4]

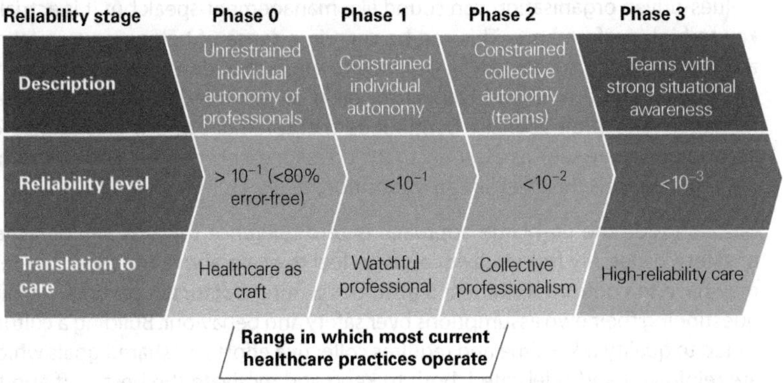

Reliability stage	Phase 0	Phase 1	Phase 2	Phase 3
Description	Unrestrained individual autonomy of professionals	Constrained individual autonomy	Constrained collective autonomy (teams)	Teams with strong situational awareness
Reliability level	$> 10^{-1}$ (<80% error-free)	$<10^{-1}$	$<10^{-2}$	$<10^{-3}$
Translation to care	Healthcare as craft	Watchful professional	Collective professionalism	High-reliability care

Range in which most current healthcare practices operate

As an organisation progresses to a state of high reliability each of these building blocks has to develop and link with the others, which is no small task even for the most renowned organisations. Yet the predominant culture within many providers is one of individual professional autonomy, where clinical excellence is the sole preserve of doctors while boards have little influence over quality. The result is that avoidable errors occur, outcomes are variable and patients are harmed. Poor quality is either undetected or tolerated as the norm.

Conversely, once safety and clinical excellence are prioritised and responsibility for quality shifts from individuals to multifunctional teams, outcomes improve dramatically and harm rates decline. High-reliability organisations typically experience errors in less than 0.5 per cent of care processes, compared with a figure elsewhere of 20 per cent.[5] As the table below shows, even at relatively high levels of reliability, the complexity of healthcare processes means that small error rates compound to create failures of much higher frequency.

	Base error rate of each step			
No. of steps				
1	0.05	0.01	0.001	0.0001
5	0.33	0.05	0.005	0.002
25	0.72	0.22	0.02	0.003
50	0.92	0.39	0.05	0.005
100	0.99	0.63	0.1	0.01

How small errors contribute to unreliability: Even at seemingly low error rates per step, more complex processes with multiple steps have unacceptably high error rates. In healthcare, error rates run at above 1 per cent per step, evidence that organisations are not 'in control.'[6]

Building a Quality Culture

All leaders of high-reliability organisations stress the importance of developing a quality-oriented culture, not just among leaders but everywhere. Being a 'values-driven organisation' can sound like management-speak but it is actually key to high performance. This can be seen in a sense of belonging to a team, a drive to excel, a constructive approach to errors that does not seek to blame individuals, and a trust and respect for each other's roles, especially between managers and professionals. Continuous measurement and a clear sense of accountability are seen as essential to the drive for excellence; in poorly performing organisations they feel like an imposition.

But alongside the no-blame approach is zero tolerance towards any breaches of safety, especially from individuals who feel they are above the rules. Leaders may have to confront entrenched attitudes among doctors in particular, while questioning their own assumptions over safety and behaviour. Building a culture tuned to quality takes time and requires collective effort and shared goals which are reinforced and celebrated, both to keep and motivate the best staff and to encourage others to aspire to work there.

As with all high-performance cultures, leadership has to demonstrate an aversion to being average. The board's role is crucial: members have to overcome their traditional deference to professionals and be closely involved in defining and measuring quality and safety. Clinicians must challenge each other. Embracing the right values is every bit as important as reporting structures and dashboards and sets an example for the entire organisation.

If minor breaches of standards gradually become accepted, major failures will follow. This 'normalised deviance' has led to disasters as varied as the NASA Challenger Shuttle explosion and the UK's Mid Staffordshire Hospital scandal. These organisations' internal processes indicated they were not doing too badly, but concealed the fact that no one was prepared to ask awkward questions.

Data has to be meaningful and actionable. Hospitals need clear outcome reporting systems and everyone needs to know who is responsible for doing what in response; even the best metrics are of little value without a clear vision of how to use them. Successful healthcare organisations no longer develop measures from the top down because they recognise that frontline staff know what is most important to track.

At University Hospitals Birmingham, UK, teams across the organisation are assigned ownership of each part of a patient pathway; there is timely monitoring and measurement of their actions and their clear accountability drives them to improve. When these owners – professionals and managers – are accountable for their performance, the organisation has the basis for continuous quality and cost improvement. The board sets the tone by making outcomes the most important objective, overseeing the design and implementation of the quality strategy and holding the chief executive and directors to account.

In the Helios hospital chain in Germany, data is reported from each clinic's medical director to the regional level and then up to headquarters. This picked up that they were scoring 'average' on stroke outcomes, which was unacceptable, so the leadership went into the best and worst clinics, learned what did and did not work and improved overall performance. Changes are often simple, such as universal adoption of the 'stroke box', which ensures that all material needed for acute stroke treatment – syringe, antithrombotic drug and checklist – is in one place. This automates the process and increases compliance with the guidelines.

When Helios takes action over performance everyone has to participate; agreed quality measures such as safe-surgery checklists are rigorously enforced, everyone in the organisation knows who is responsible for doing what and there is a clear message that anyone who does not comply with 'must dos' will be out.

The Central Role of Standardisation

Standardisation is key to reliability. When every surgeon uses his or her preferred technique irrespective of the wider clinical team there is a higher chance of errors. In a high-reliability organisation, on the other hand, measurement, roles and culture are all aligned with standard pathways and operating procedures which reduce complexity and variation, improve cooperation and communication and enhance quality. With a higher level of scrutiny and checks, processes become far more resilient. Frontline staff are responsible for confirming that guidelines are being followed and have the capability and will to intervene if they believe this is not happening.

In Utah in the US, standardisation has delivered dramatic and continuous improvements for Intermountain Healthcare. It is one of the pioneers of integrating standard processes with measurement of outcomes and its rigorous approach has ensured that guidelines that could have soon been forgotten have instead become automated pathways – the default way of doing things. Workflows throughout the hospital, from the bedside to the operating theatre, are built around standardised processes.

For Intermountain patients seriously ill with acute respiratory distress syndrome, the rate of guideline variances dropped from 59 per cent to 6 per cent within four months.[7] Patient survival increased from 9.5 per cent to 44 per cent, physicians' time commitments fell by about half and the total cost of care decreased by a quarter. This approach has since been extended to 104 clinical processes that account for the vast majority of Intermountain's care, with similar success. The group is now widely regarded as one of the top providers in the US, achieving excellent outcomes at low cost.

There is a history of deep resistance among doctors towards standardisation. But the best physicians recognise that it goes hand in hand with clinical expertise and judgement, which can now be focused on the unique aspects of any given case.

An Obsession With Measurement

The best organisations are obsessed with measurement. At the Mayo Clinic in the US, state-of-the-art internal dashboards are commonplace from the ward up, measuring outcomes, prevention practices, re-admissions, length of stay, throughput time and compliance with protocols. Many measures are fed automatically in real-time to staff and, where appropriate, managers and the board. Data is fed back to the owners of clinical pathways to drive continuous improvement.

High reliability is, inevitably, more of a journey than a destination. The starting point may be that care is excellent but not consistently so, with no effective board oversight of quality and a lack of control over clinical risks. Outcomes are not uniformly measured or reported and quality is not central to the culture. Responsibility for outcomes is poorly defined, with few protocols centred around patients.

In the first stage of the high-reliability journey, safety and clinical excellence become part of the organisation's priorities, along with a growing understanding that progress is dependent upon systems rather than individuals. Measurement of outcomes becomes more common but not yet standard and attention to quality is more systematic, from the board down to the ground floor, with higher adherence to protocols and checklists.

Only the most advanced organisations reach the next stage, where key outcomes and their drivers are routinely measured and reported and aligned with the board's quality objectives. The culture is intolerant of breaking basic rules while taking a blame-free learning approach to errors. Teams have clear responsibility for care pathways and monitor the impact of their performance on patient outcomes.

For the few organisations that succeed in marshalling all this work to achieve high-reliability care, preventing failures becomes the leading drive. This 'failsafe' approach will be focused on high-risk environments such as operating rooms and emergency departments.

Becoming a high-reliability organisation is a big ambition – but the public demands it and the business case for those delivering, receiving or contracting care is clear. Ultimately, delivering high-quality care is why most providers and staff went into healthcare in the first place.

Focusing on the Irrelevant and Unreliable

As payers, patients, governments and regulators demand to know more about care delivery and quality, many executives I meet comment on the tension between how they feel their organisation should be held to account and how their health systems actually judge them. There is overwhelming concern that the increasing number of measures imposed on providers are largely irrelevant and even harmful. While acknowledging the rights of patients and payers to know the outcomes that matter to them, managers and clinicians feel that the incessant demands for information from regulators, state and federal governments, accreditation agencies and professional bodies can impede transparency and accountability rather than encourage it. Being compelled to measure the wrong things is more than just an irritation; it sends out confusing, distracting and demotivating messages to employees which diminish staff engagement and can even undermine the authority of the board.

My hope is that over the next few years measurement will increasingly become standardised internationally as providers, payers and governments acknowledge the need to converge around the outcomes that matter to patients. This will accelerate the sharing of knowledge and innovation around the globe.

Professionals and researchers are used to discussing those outcomes – known as 'primary endpoints' – that matter to patients. In stroke care, for example, the status 90 days after the onset of stroke is seen as the primary outcome measure on the road to optimum recovery. For rheumatoid arthritis patients the most important intermediate goal – a strong predictor of long-term outcomes – is controlling the disease activity, as measured by a few questions and a blood test. Once hospitals are able to measure and report these outcomes reliably and demonstrate improvements over time, there should be no need to publicly report a plethora of process and intermediate measures.

This is a new approach and the sector is still trying to define the key outcomes and find ways to measure them. But there are promising signs. In oncology and cardiovascular surgery, standardised outcome measures are becoming available through internationally coordinated clinical registries, while the Dutch health insurers' association has worked with leading doctors to use its all-payer database to establish key outcome measures for conditions such as strokes and Parkinson's disease.

However, if stakeholders are to act on and pay for the reported outcomes, the measures need to be reliable. Data is often not gathered in a standardised way, while systems used for recording and reporting are typically unsophisticated and lack the kind of double-entry facility seen in the accounts. Consequently most publicly reported outcome data is still unreliable, especially when compared with the internal and external controls which assure the accuracy of healthcare organisations' finances.

In the rush to request data, governments, payers and regulators are often failing to question whether reports can be trusted. Indeed, there have been cases where data has been altered to improve scores; in the Netherlands the breast cancer recurrence scores reported by some hospitals were lower than the numbers sent to the clinical registries. Such 'gaming' becomes more common when professionals and providers question the point of collecting the data.

The Hospital Standardised Mortality Rate (HSMR) is another example of questionable reliability and 'gaming' undermining validity. It was developed over a decade ago to capture the quality of a hospital in a single number. The HSMR looks at the number of people that die in a hospital in relation to the number of people that would be expected to die, taking into consideration the case-mix of patients. The validity of HSMR has increasingly been challenged, partly due to coding differences that create large fluctuations in the score and partly because of the huge variation in patients and care in different hospitals. Yet the UK, for example, still publishes scores prominently and hospitals are criticised for above-average HSMR rates. Deserved scepticism can lead to hospitals massaging their figures to achieve a more desirable score.

But many organisations do value data reliability. Auditors are asked to assess the accuracy and completeness of reporting, drawing on their extensive experience with financial records. In Canada, the UK, Portugal, the US and elsewhere there are new requirements for data assurance. In the UK, all NHS providers must publish an annual set of independently checked Quality Accounts, with a director's statement confirming balance and accuracy.

Conclusion

As healthcare organisations strive to gain control over quality through the journey to high reliability, the pursuit of excellence and safety will gradually become systematic as they head towards a culture focused on outcomes, safety and measurement. Responsibility for quality will be less reliant on individuals and more on teams. Staff will embrace standardised processes, leading to improved outcomes and a sharp decline in harm.

The sleepless nights for modern healthcare leaders come from knowing enough to see the gaps. But we now have the improvement science to build high reliability into all our clinical systems. We expect it from other industries and we should expect the same high standards for ourselves and our loved ones.

References

[1] James J.T., 'A new, evidence-based estimate of patient harms associated with hospital care,' *Journal of Patient Safety*, 9 (3), pp. 122–8 (2013).

[2] Hogan H. et al., 'Preventable deaths due to problems in care in English acute hospitals,' *British Medical Journal Quality & Safety*, 22 (2) (2013).

[3] Department for Transport, Number of fatalities resulting from road accidents in Great Britain (UK Government, 2011).

[4] KPMG International, The more I know the less I sleep: Global perspectives on clinical governance (KPMG, 2013).

[5] Nolan T.W., 'System changes to improve patients safety,' *British Medical Journal*, 320, pp. 771–3 (2000).

[6] Ibid.

[7] KPMG International (2013).

30 Value Walks

There is no healthcare without the workforce

All over the world I have seen hospitals struggling to get the best – and the most – from their staff. Rising demand, cost pressures and chronic staff shortages in many countries mean it has never been more important to ensure staff are productive and motivated but many organisations are still getting the basics wrong.

With staff forming by far the largest cost in any healthcare system, the growing demand too often triggers a single-minded push for ever greater productivity which undermines the motivation of the very workforce needed to drive improvements. KPMG research shows that staff are frequently treated simply as a cost to the system rather than the source of its value.[1] The old mindset that 'cost walks on two legs' needs to be replaced with a new one: 'value walks'.

While many industries have benefited from the exponential growth in the processing power of digital technology – often known as Moore's Law after Intel co-founder Gordon Moore – the productivity of healthcare in developed countries has tended to lurch from increase to decrease. Industries from manufacturing to retail have centralised, standardised, upskilled and downskilled in pursuit of ever greater productivity but in healthcare we have random systems which are not focused on the needs of the customers, with poor control over the means of production.

UK healthcare is a good example. The Nuffield Trust has shown how hospital productivity in England rose by about 20 per cent between 1974 and 1999 before falling by an average of 1.4 per cent a year between 1995 and 2008, largely as a result of big spending increases from the turn of the century.[2] Since then, many nursing posts have been cut to reduce costs, before being reintroduced to address shortcomings in quality.

The widening gap between the rapidly growing demand for health services and a steady decline in the health workers to service it is a global phenomenon. KPMG analysis shows that by 2022 the OECD countries will be facing a workforce shortfall of somewhere around 22–29 per cent.[3] Meanwhile the 2008 economic crash has constrained the ability of Western countries to hire the staff they need.

Running Faster, Cutting Harder

There is a strong temptation for managers and system leaders to try to solve their productivity problems by pushing everyone to run faster while cutting the workforce. But while the current financial climate has led many organisations to opt for quick fixes through cuts, the reality is that in the long run mass redundancies in healthcare almost always turn out to be unproductive. Telling staff to see more patients every day can diminish quality, increase errors, reduce workforce satisfaction and staff retention and drive up absenteeism. There is also considerable evidence that cost-cutting in a way which is unsustainable soon results in costs bouncing back into the system.

In terms of supply, demographic trends such as an ageing population and shrinking workforce in the West do not mean that the inevitable destiny is a massive workforce shortage. Many factors are at play, such as levels of immigration and changes in clinical practice. Attracting staff from overseas has bolstered numbers in developed countries from Britain to Australia, but it is controversial. Often it simply relocates shortages to less-developed countries where wages are lower while stripping the home economy of expensively trained and badly needed personnel.

There are many policies that could bridge the healthcare workforce gap.[4] For example, if all OECD countries shared Japan's high retirement age and Greece's long working hours they could enjoy a 35 per cent gain in labour capacity. The gap could also be closed if more women were brought into the healthcare workforce: differences in female participation rates are substantial and could represent a 10 per cent labour capacity gain if the average OECD country achieved northern European levels. Significant variations between OECD countries also emerge when comparing the size of the healthcare workforce as a share of total employment. The average share for OECD countries is 10 per cent, with Greece down at 5 per cent and Norway up at 20 per cent, leaving considerable room for growth. So one way or another the predicted workforce gap of 22–29 per cent can be closed. The problem is that Western countries cannot endlessly throw money at the problem to pay for more staff.

In the developing world the problem is even more severe. WHO estimates that some 57 African and Asian countries will soon face a critical shortage of healthcare workers but will not have the economies to allow them to spend their way out.[5]

The challenge, therefore, is to close the potential workforce gap in a new and radical way: by enhancing the productivity of healthcare personnel while at the same time improving the quality of care and the attractiveness of the work. Across the world, systems that have achieved this tend to share five characteristics: a strategic focus on value for patients, empowered professionals, intelligent process redesign, effective use of management information, and management of staff performance.

Patient Value

Many physicians see the term 'value' as a euphemism for cost-cutting. Nevertheless, an increasing number of organisations now see enhancing value for patients – in other words, concentrating on what matters to them – as a fundamental goal. Putting patient value at the heart of the system is the first step to unlocking higher quality, lower costs and better productivity.

Ensuring healthcare organisations have a strong sense of what matters to patients means it is much more likely that clinicians and managers will share goals, which in turn makes difficult conversations about issues such as performance and the redesign of work processes easier and more constructive. Successful organisations embed the search for value for patients in everything they do – goal-setting, strategy, management information, recruitment methods, reward systems and staff behaviour.

In the Netherlands, the Buurtzorg (meaning neighbourhood care) home care organisation provides a powerful example of how to provide value for patients while giving staff more autonomy, raising productivity and cutting costs. Dutch home care is highly fragmented with various tasks – such as washing the patient and changing dressings – paid through different reimbursement schemes and usually executed by different staff. As a result, care lacks coordination, making it difficult to respond to a patient's changing condition. At the same time, many service providers have cut costs by fine-tuning the minimum skill level required for each task. So care tends to respond to patients' current problems rather than preventing deterioration.

Buurtzorg empowers nurses (rather than nursing assistants or domestic staff) to deliver all the care that patients need. It hires better experienced (and more expensive) staff but operates a remarkably flat structure: the 8,000 nurses are supported by fewer than 50 back-office staff and very few managers.[6] While this has meant higher costs per hour, the result has been fewer hours in total. By changing the model of care, Buurtzorg has cut the number of care hours by half, improved quality and raised staff satisfaction. In 2011 it was chosen as Dutch employer of the year.

The nurses organise their own work and use their professional expertise to solve patients' problems by making the most of their clients' capabilities to become more self-sufficient. Simply put, Buurtzorg nurses aim to make themselves superfluous as soon as possible. Patient satisfaction scores are 30 per cent above the national average and the number of episodes requiring costly unplanned interventions has dropped.[7] If the entire Dutch home care system operated on this level of effectiveness it would free up somewhere in the region of 7,000 full-time staff.

Responsible Autonomy

The lesson from Buurtzorg is that staff are most likely to be productive if they feel empowered. Command and control methods do not work well in complex environments; staff with limited discretion are less able to solve problems, identify improvements or exercise initiative. Worse, low levels of autonomy have been found to undermine recruitment and retention and increase patient mortality.[8]

Empowering staff means giving them freedom to manage their own work while encouraging a desire to get better at what they do and promoting a sense of purpose about why they are doing it. If professionals are to be in the lead they need to learn team-working, leadership and improvement skills and be coached and supported as they learn.

Empowering staff gives them a personal responsibility for driving improvement. Clinicians have told me on countless occasions about how they want to be more productive, but claim they are being held back by 'the system'. In effect, they are sitting back and waiting for everything else to be fixed before they make their move. This organisational inertia should not be tolerated.

Crucially, there needs to be a discussion between managers and doctors about what is expected and how staff will be held to account. This is a change from the traditional relationship between physicians and their employers; in the past autonomy has been interpreted as the freedom to practise medicine unconstrained by cost considerations and with little accountability. Managers typically lack the confidence – and indeed the courage – to provide leadership to clinicians, which allows the status quo to prevail. Now a new model of responsible autonomy needs to be negotiated in which professionals are given the power to do a better job and are held to account for the outcomes. But this autonomy does not extend to perpetuating the random systems which currently beset healthcare providers. Instead, staff need to work to agreed, evidence-based care pathways and procedures, with decisions to depart from them recorded and discussed.

Without the active engagement of doctors, organisations have no chance of implementing radical improvements. The problem in many places is that changing expectations of doctors, coupled with increased accountability and requirements to work more systematically, have challenged their traditional relationship with the hospital. The privileges that doctors have enjoyed, such as a high level of freedom and toleration of behaviours not permitted in other

Virginia Mason Medical Center in Seattle is well known for its application of the Toyota production system to healthcare, but its work in changing the relationship between the organisation and its doctors – the human side of the system – is just as impressive. For example, it organised a retreat for physicians and managers which gave physicians the opportunity to talk candidly about their frustrations and the sense of loss of autonomy and entitlement. The retreat gave managers and physicians the chance to debate what a new compact between the organisation and its staff should look like. This, in turn, triggered months of work involving a broad group encompassing both enthusiasts and sceptics. Department meetings were held in which the draft compact was discussed, revised and eventually approved. The final document established reciprocal expectations between Virginia Mason and its physicians. A few chose to leave but the widespread support for the compact meant that both parties shared a vision of Virginia Mason as a quality leader in healthcare. This unity of purpose enabled the medical centre's ambitious improvement programmes to succeed.

Gary Kaplan MD, president and CEO of Virginia Mason, reflects that it was essential to be transparent about everything the organisation was trying to do: where it was, where it was trying to get to, what it expected of its staff and what staff could expect of the organisation. That was the only way to ensure its physicians bought into the values of the organisation and felt motivated. He has used a Japanese word – nemawashi – to capture why the compact was so successful. It means 'tilling the soil', which in this context refers to taking the time to have deep conversations.

staff, are now under attack. But the old deal is being replaced without an explicit conversation; across the world this has been manifesting itself in discontent among doctors.

The antidote is to discuss openly with physicians what is changing and why, and then create a shared vision and an explicit deal that supports both the organisation's success and physicians' professional satisfaction. This approach is based on research around the idea of the 'psychological contract'.

Many of the most radical initiatives in empowering staff can be seen in developing countries such as Mozambique, which is critically short of healthcare workers.[9] After independence in 1975 there were 80 doctors to serve a population of 14 million and hardly any staff capable of providing emergency obstetric care. In 1984 it began exploring a new approach to staff empowerment, training non-medical staff in obstetric surgery.

While obstetric surgery is traditionally conducted by gynaecologists, many obstetric surgical interventions, such as caesarean sections, can be performed by trained non-physicians. The country began to recruit healthcare workers from rural areas to take on this role. Candidates had to have at least a three-year degree as a nurse or a medical assistant and then complete a two-year course which was followed by an internship with a surgeon. Successful recruits become 'tecnicos de cirurgia', a role comparable to surgically trained assistant medical officer.

The tecnicos have become a vital part of rural obstetric care. Staff retention rates are high; in one study 88 per cent were still working in the countryside seven years after graduation, compared with a seven-year retention rate for rural physicians of zero.[10] Decision-making and quality of care, gauged by indicators such as post-operative deaths and major complications, are comparable to obstetricians. The tecnicos initiative is exceptionally cost-effective: training one tecnico costs US$19,465, compared with US$74,130 for a physician.

But while there are many opportunities to shift tasks to lower-paid and less extensively trained staff it is a mistake to assume that this is always the answer. In emergency care, for example, having the most skilled and experienced decision-maker as early in the process as possible produces better results and lower costs, while Buurtzorg in the Netherlands shows the power of upskilling.

Standardisation and Systematic Redesign

Many tasks and processes in healthcare have more to do with tradition and staff convenience than patients' needs. Improving efficiency through the standardisation and systematic redesign of care is a key habit of successful organisations. The best embed continuous improvement in their work alongside more radical redesign of staff roles and processes. Although improved efficiency may mean seeing more patients, it can increase job satisfaction by removing the pointless work staff have to do to fix broken systems, look for missing equipment or deal with failure to get care right first time.

Clinical pathways are at the heart of system redesign. They enable the right skills to be matched to the task, the elimination of waste, the minimisation of variation and risk, and the engagement of clinical staff in design and improvement. Leading organisations have started to treat knowledge management as a major organisational competence, designing best practice into processes rather than having to rely on hiring the most knowledgeable individuals.

The Aravind Eye Care System in India is a celebrated example of process redesign. Ophthalmologist Dr Govindappa Venkataswamy founded a clinic in 1976 with just 11 beds. Today Aravind is the world's largest provider of eye care services, treating more than 2.6 million outpatients and performing more than

300,000 ophthalmic high-volume surgeries every year. Its mission is to eliminate preventable blindness; India is home to 9 million of the world's 45 million blind people.

The system enables doctors to be as productive as possible by limiting their responsibilities to diagnoses, verifying test results and performing surgery using an assembly-line approach. Care quality is monitored extensively and reported transparently. The clinics follow a 'no-secrets' rule where complication rates are presented monthly by clinic as well as by individual surgeon, allowing the leaders to drive improvements. Aravind optimises the flow of patients through the clinics, resulting in faster throughput times and fewer patient visits. Its doctors achieve world-class outcomes while performing an average of 2,000 operations every year, compared with 400 by other Indian doctors.

The Power of Data

Aravind shows the power of data in improving workforce productivity. The best organisations collect data about processes and outcomes, which can be used to drive improvement. Data enables them to test improvement ideas, develop their knowledge about what works and change their practice. This requires staff that are clear about value, empowered and trained to make improvements and have the tools to specify and design high-quality care. Measurement and feedback reinforce this culture of improvement. The end point is to steer the organisation by outcomes – for example measuring infection rates rather than adherence to hand hygiene policy. There is some way to go before this is the norm.

Getting the Management Right

Human resource management in many healthcare organisations is transactional, traditional, risk averse, lacking strategic perspective and rarely prepared to challenge current practice. While the high performing organisations I have discussed embrace innovation, they also appreciate that these initiatives must be built on a platform of good staff management. Failure in this area can fatally undermine staff commitment to the values of the organisation and support for its leadership. Wherever I go in the world, I often ask groups of hospital staff if they have had an appraisal in the past year, I rarely see more than a third of hands go up. This is not the way to show staff they are valued, nor is it the best way to encourage discretionary effort.

Good management must start at the recruitment stage by ensuring staff not only have the right skills but understand and support the organisation's values. The recruitment of people who are resilient in the face of change is important.

Induction into the organisation must be taken seriously. Staff need clearly defined roles supported by systems for ensuring they get high-quality feedback and appraisals which are linked to rewards and based on meaningful metrics. As well as recognising good performance, the best organisations are rigorous about dealing with poor performance, behaviour at odds with their values and absenteeism. A willingness to let staff go who do not measure up to the organisation's values is essential; failure to do so sends the message that the values are optional.

Conclusion

Taken together, the five measures I have discussed here – a strategic focus on value for patients, empowered staff, process redesign, effective use of information, and management of staff performance – can enable providers to outperform their peers in quality of care, attractiveness of work and productivity. There is a strong ethical and business imperative to do this. All these measures need to be executed together, rigorously and continuously. If done well they have the potential to buy healthcare organisations enough time and staff support for more fundamental changes to their business and care models, of which the innovations here are just the beginning. If change is a human contact sport, we had best contact human beings.

References

1 KPMG International, Value walks: Successful habits for improving workforce motivation (KPMG, 2013).

2 Hurst J. and Williams S., Can NHS hospitals do more with less? (Nuffield Trust, 2012).

3 KPMG International (2013), p. 7.

4 KPMG International (2013), p. 11.

5 Global Health Workforce Alliance Statistics (World Health Organization, 2009).

6 KPMG International, Staying power: Stories of success in global healthcare (KPMG, 2014).

7 KPMG International (2013), p. 20.

8 West M. et al., 'Reducing patient mortality in hospitals: The role of human resource management,' *Journal of Organizational Behaviour*, (27), pp. 983–1002 (2006).

9 KPMG International (2013), p. 28.

10 Kruk, M. et al., 'Economic evaluation of surgically trained assistant medical officers in performing major obstetric surgery in Mozambique' in *British Journal of Obstetrics and Gynaecology*, (114), pp.1253–60 (2007).

31 Patients As Partners

Renewable energy

Healthcare systems across the world are struggling to secure more money and more staff while failing to exploit the one resource they have in abundance: patients. Health systems that truly partner with patients will find abundant sources of renewable energy.

The alignment between what patients want and what they get is often poor. The goals of patients are not given enough recognition in treatment choices and the benefits of shared decision-making and patient and carer empowerment are not being realised.

I suspect that my experience of being diagnosed with prostate cancer at the age of 42 reflects that of many patients who suddenly discover they have a serious illness. Initially, the only 'empowerment' I was interested in was having the cancer removed. Yet within three weeks I went from being fit and able to having a radical prostatectomy and I was left incontinent, infertile and impotent. Fortunately two of these three problems were reversed over time but the physical discomfort was nothing compared with the psychological distress. It is not uncommon for cancer patients to feel low or depressed and I certainly felt alone with no one to talk to.

The technical side of my care was world class and saved my life but it was not matched by the post-operative support. Once I had left hospital – the day of the operation – there was little ongoing care, and poor communication with the community team and my GP left me as the care coordinator, a task I took on as an enthusiastic amateur.

On reflection, I think if people had helped me become a partner in my care then I would have been better prepared for the emotional and physical side effects and made a quicker recovery. As it was, I didn't know who to turn to. I remember seeing a cancer helpdesk in the hospital open from 10am to 2pm – hardly convenient for my work or flexible enough for most patients. I wanted to help other patients like me and joined the board of Prostate Cancer UK to try to make a difference. All of my royalties for this book will be donated to the organisation and the excellent work they do.

Technically Good, Emotionally Poor

My experience chimes with many of the messages we received from patients around the world when KPMG conducted a global survey of 27 patient groups in six countries across four continents. Time and again, people said that while the technical side of their care was good, there were particular transition points where they felt 'abandoned' and where their health may have suffered as a result. Post-diagnosis was a particularly vulnerable point but discharge from acute and specialist care was also highlighted. Overall, patients recognised the difficult job that healthcare workers face – and were grateful to them – but around the world the message came back to recognise and value the assets and abilities that patients can bring to their care, to treat them as people rather than 'sites for intervention', to communicate information better and to share decision-making.

This failure to take advantage of 'people power' is another example of healthcare being slow to learn from other industries. As customers in banking and retail sectors, we now routinely take responsibility for tasks that staff used to do for us and value the control and flexibility this brings. But few healthcare organisations invest any real training resource into their patients.

As a recent global study by the UK Parliament observes, patient empowerment is increasingly being recognised as a solution to many of the most pressing problems facing healthcare, including the growing burden of chronic diseases, the need to encourage healthier lifestyles and the challenge of coordinating care for people with multiple conditions.[1] A powerful evidence base now exists to demonstrate how patient involvement can lead to improved patient experience, understanding, behaviours and safety, as well as reduced use of services.[2]

Dignity, Respect and Safety

Patient power is not only efficient by improving the outcomes that matter to patients and allowing new models of care to be created, it reflects core values of dignity, respect and safety. It is a recognition that patients, carers and communities all have particular needs and aspirations. Embedding this culture requires a sophisticated understanding of the attitudes, desires and characteristics of individual patients, groups of patients and communities, with the goals of everyone from the leadership to the clinical teams concentrating on creating high-quality outcomes and experiences for those patients. This, in turn, requires a culture of continuous improvement and a decisive move away from organising goals around the work of teams or departments rather than the overall value created for the patient's journey.

Many organisations think they are already empowering patients, but patients themselves overwhelmingly say they are not. Two attitudes are getting in the way: empowering patients has been viewed as the 'right thing to do' rather than crucial to the economic sustainability of healthcare systems, so it has not been pursued with any urgency; and clinicians are wary of the idea because it changes the power relationship between them and their patients.

Many of the world's best consumer-facing companies design their products this way and some healthcare providers are trying to do likewise. Some use a story built around a typical patient as a way of helping staff understand what they need to do to put the patient at the centre of their work. In Jönköping County in Sweden, staff created Esther, an elderly woman with a chronic illness, as a way to mobilise change such as better care coordination and patient flows. This has become so integral to how the system works that parts of the patient pathway are now named after her; Esther coaches – usually nursing assistants – are charged with helping to bring the patient perspective into daily practice.

Involving Patients in Service Design

Organisations need to involve patients and carers in designing services to understand how they perceive the different parts of healthcare and what value they receive from them. Talking to patients helps to identify steps that should be removed, which improves the patient experience while driving up productivity. There are many ways of using the experiences of patients and carers in service design, such as interviews, observations, diaries, stories and ethnography.

Involving patients in design should not be seen as an extra layer of checks. On the contrary, it is a different way of thinking about teams, organisations, structures, flows, productivity and outcomes. Analysing the system through the eyes of the patient will challenge clinical hierarchies, question the value of different skills and overturn long-established patterns of behaviour. It is difficult work which takes time to get right, but it can have a profound effect on patient experience, care quality and system efficiency.

So-called 'preference misdiagnosis' is another important lens through which to view patient power, since it represents a clear 'lose-lose' scenario of waste for the system and poor care for the patient. Dr Albert Mulley, Director of the Dartmouth Center for Health Care Delivery Science in the US, believes there is a widespread failure by clinicians to understand their patients' preferences and how proposed interventions will affect their lives. There is also growing concern in some countries about 'over-diagnosis' in which patients are over-investigated and screened and sometimes harmed. Patients who are fully informed about their options often make decisions which are more conservative and lower cost than the course recommended by their physician, which means they are more likely to get an outcome with which they are happy while saving the system money. For example, patient decision aids have been shown to reduce the need for elective procedures by 21 per cent while delivering an improved experience and equal health outcomes.[3]

One of the barriers to patient empowerment is that many clinicians support the idea but feel they don't have the time. It takes investment and training to give staff the skills to help patients understand their condition and treatment options and to express their preferences. Health coaches are needed to work alongside patients, provide decision aids and document preferences.

The Language of Compliance

The common decision by patients not to take prescribed medication is a measure of the gap between them and their clinicians when it comes to having a shared understanding of treatment goals. It is thought that between a third and a half of all medicines prescribed for long-term conditions are not taken as recommended.[4] This is a major source of inadequate outcomes and costs healthcare systems dearly. One estimate in the US in 2009 put the total cost of this outcome at $290 billion, or 13 per cent of total healthcare spending.

But clinicians talk about the problem in the language of 'compliance' or 'adherence', betraying how little thought has been given to the patient as a consumer of services and medicines. No consumer-orientated industry would expect its customers to 'comply' with its wishes – they have an approach that recognises the power of the consumer over their own choices.

The National Institute of Health and Care Excellence in the UK has recognised that if patients are to take their drugs they need to be more involved in discussions with their GP about the drugs themselves. In 2009 it issued new guidelines for involving patients when prescribing, pointing out that: 'Medicine-taking is a complex human behaviour, and patients evaluate medicines and the risks and benefits of medicines according to the resources available to them. Unwanted and unused medicines reflect inadequate communication between professionals and patients about health problems and how they might be treated.'[5]

Finding ways to improve patient understanding of drug therapies, such as by coaching them in how a drug works, how it affects the disease and interacts with other medication, and the consequences of not taking it, would be one of the most effective ways of improving the value of the medicines themselves while aligning the decisions of the clinician with the interests of the patient.

End-of-life care is perhaps the area where shared decision-making can have the greatest impact on both patients and the health economy. A characteristic of high-quality, high-productivity organisations is that they take the trouble to help patients plan ahead, including for the end of their life. Clinicians can incur high costs in pursuit of futile and often distressing care for dying patients simply because they did not have the right conversations beforehand.

Self-care

But clinicians informing and involving patients is only half the story. For most patients, for most of their illness, the people who put the greatest time and effort into caring for them are themselves and their family or carer. Patients need to manage their condition for about 5,800 waking hours each year while typically spending fewer than 10 hours with a healthcare professional.[6] Yet only a small minority of those professionals have recognised how they can increase the value of self-care. This is untapped renewable energy.

Investing in the skills and capabilities of patients, carers and communities to support self-management is a challenge for traditional providers and payers. It may involve new skills and roles, such as coaching and motivational interviewing, and new ways of engaging with patients to identify the resources they have and to develop the options available to them. 'Social prescribing' – signposting patients to non-healthcare services such as community groups to reduce social isolation – also becomes important.

Supporting patients in looking after themselves needs to become a core skill for healthcare organisations. There are numerous channels to support self-diagnosis and management, such as phone and online services, pharmacies and community workers, while apps, decision aids and care navigators can help patients find their way through the system.

Perhaps the boldest approach to this I have encountered is the Care Companion programme developed by Narayana Health in India.[7] Here, the carers of at-risk patients are taken aside during an admission and given a short course in post-operative care and support, initially through interactive videos and classroom demonstrations and then supervised on the hospital wards. This allows patients to be better cared for when they leave the hospital and less likely to require re-admission. It also helps to build the confidence and skills of carers to manage their loved one at home and know when further professional care is and is not needed.

The Economic Case for Activated Patients

There is compelling evidence that so-called 'patient activation' like this reduces costs. A study in the US indicated that patients with the least skills and confidence to engage in their own care cost between 8 per cent and 21 per cent more than the most 'activated' patients.[8] The important lesson here is that healthcare staff should aim to use every interaction with a patient to increase their capacity to be active in their own care, such as by growing their understanding of the condition or encouraging them to make lifestyle changes. The researchers recommended that providers should monitor patient activation scores to encourage more patient engagement as a way of improving outcomes and cutting costs. The tool used to conduct this study – the Patient Activation Measure (PAM) – has now been translated into 22 languages and has the potential to become a transferrable indicator for international comparisons of improving patient involvement – something the world is long overdue.[9]

Predicted per capita costs of patients by patient activation level[10]

2010 patient activation level	Predicted per capita billed costs ($)	Ratio of predicted costs relative to level 4 Patient Activation Measure (PAM)
Level 1 (lowest)	966	1.21
Level 2	840	1.05
Level 3	783	0.97
Level 4 (highest)	799	1.00

One new trend in providing information is 'gamification' – using games to engage patients. The potential is immense; computer, tablet and mobile phone games can encourage goal-setting, support adherence to treatment, develop cognitive or motor skills, provide education, and support forms of self-care such as exercising and diet management. Some games even introduce elements of collaboration and rivalry between groups of patients, for example in lifestyle changes. I have seen this work well in American companies who pay for their own health insurance and run employee wellness programmes.

Influencing Research

Patient power is also beginning to influence research. At present, there is limited evidence that patients' views are making much impact on the shape of programmes but this will have to change in a world in which patient value will increasingly become part of the decision-making process for research investment. The Seventh Framework Programme (FP7), the

EU's current research-funding system, stresses the importance of patient and public involvement, while the Patient-Centered Outcomes Research Institute in Washington DC has allocated US$68 million to a research network predicated on the principle that 'the interests of patients will be central to decision-making'.[11]

The opportunities for engaging patients in research are being explored by less conventional actors such as Shift MS, which brings young people with multiple sclerosis together, and PatientsLikeMe, a patient network where people connect with others who have the same disease or condition and track and share their own experiences. In the process, they generate data about the disease that helps researchers, purchasers and providers develop more effective treatments.

Low-tech and 'no-tech' solutions to patient empowerment are also being found by less-developed economies, often in response to critical shortages of health workers. Countries such as Bangladesh, India, Malawi and Nepal have found that the simple intervention of getting groups of local women together to discuss for themselves how to reduce maternal and newborn deaths has led to dramatic improvements in health. Self-directed and using participatory methods such as voting, role-play and storytelling, the groups showed reductions in maternal and neonatal mortality of 37 per cent and 23 per cent respectively in a trial covering over 100,000 births.[12] If this were a drug it would make headlines around the world; why should a patient involvement intervention be any different?

Conclusion

Implicit in all these approaches is that healthcare organisations and staff cede power to patients and communities and start to implement new ways of working. But patient power is not a zero-sum game. It is a win-win. Leaders need to create a culture where patient experience is continually measured and improved and where concerns and complaints are learned from and welcomed. Hospital boards should be aware of complaints and key quality concerns and the actions being taken to address them. Data created by clinical teams needs to be fed back rapidly and used to identify trends and solutions. Patient experience needs to be at the heart of staff appraisals.

The benefits of using patient power to improve value and quality are immense and largely untapped. It is time all healthcare systems released the power of patients, families and communities to improve the quality and experience of care and reduce costs. As the greatest untapped resource in healthcare, patient power will increasingly be the factor that makes our health systems sustainable.

References

[1] All-Party Parliamentary Group on Global Health, Patient empowerment: For better quality more sustainable health services globally (APPG-GH, 2014).

[2] Coulter A. and Ellins J., 'Effectiveness of strategies for informing, educating, and involving patients,' *British Medical Journal*, 335, pp. 24–7 (2007).

[3] Stacey D. et al., 'Decision aids for people facing treatment or screening decisions,' Cochrane Database of Systematic Reviews, 1, p. CD001431 (2014).

[4] National Institute for Health and Care Excellence, NICE Guideline CG76: Medicines adherence involving patients in decisions about prescribed medicines and supporting adherence (NICE, 2009).

[5] NICE (2009).

[6] Department of Health, Research evidence on the effectiveness of self-care support (DH, 2007).

[7] APPG Global Health (2014), p. 14.

[8] Hibbard J.H. et al., 'Patients with lower activation associated with higher costs: Delivery systems should know their patients' "scores",' *Health Affairs*, 32, pp. 216–22 (2013).

[9] Hibbard J.H. (2013).

[10] Ibid.

[11] http://www.pcori.org.

[12] Prost et al., 'Women's groups practicing participatory learning and action to improve maternal and newborn health in low-resource settings: A systematic review and meta-analysis,' *The Lancet*, 18, 381 (9879), pp. 1736–46 (2013).

32 Climate Change and Sustainability

Our dirty little secret

As someone who has managed a hospital, a region and a national health service, I understand the pressure to focus on short-term problems at the expense of long-term goals. I certainly don't think of myself as a natural climate-change champion but I am now convinced that transformed models of care can, and should, be good for people and the planet. For example, if all health systems across the planet modernised their combined heat and power facilities the world would inhale fewer emissions and health organisations would be financially better off.

This might sound rich coming from someone who flies so frequently that I am on my fourth passport in six years, but I agree with *The Lancet* when it says that climate change is 'the greatest global health threat of the twenty-first century',[1] and the hidden contribution of the healthcare sector is our dirty little secret. I have included climate change as one of the key themed chapters for this book not only because of the magnitude of the threat to human health but also because it is so intertwined with the other problems facing healthcare around the world. At its core, global warming is just one more outcome of the potentially unsustainable path healthcare is taking, along with spiralling costs, a focus on treatment at the expense of prevention and continued investment into models of care that no longer fit the population's needs. It adds yet more weight to the case for change and forces leaders to take the long-term development of their health system much more seriously.

There can now be little serious doubt of the reality of human-induced global warming. Scientific consensus of the link between greenhouse gas emissions and climate change only grows stronger and the effects – once hypothetical risks in the future – are already becoming a clear and present danger in the form of rising sea levels, increasingly unpredictable weather patterns, extreme weather events and volatile energy markets. We used to have to imagine these effects; now we only need to read the news.

The Role of Healthcare in Global Warming

What is less visible is the significant role that healthcare plays in causing this slow-motion train crash. Across the EU, healthcare accounts for around 5 per cent of greenhouse gas emissions, equivalent to that of the international aviation and shipping industries combined.[2] In the US this figure is thought to be as much as 8 per cent, making it the second most energy-intensive sector after fast food.[3]

Few systems have dug beneath these figures in detail but England is one. The NHS Sustainable Development Unit has been conducting a comprehensive carbon footprint exercise since 2008. This has generated valuable data about the scale of healthcare's emissions – and some counter-intuitive findings about which areas are the most polluting.

For example, the NHS is a major source of the nation's road traffic with around 5 per cent of vehicle emissions coming from related transport (patients, staff and supplies).[4] As the table below shows, however, the things healthcare providers buy – above all drugs and medical supplies – are by far the biggest contributor, almost double that of direct electricity and fuel use combined.[5]

NHS, Public Health and Social Care carbon footprint breakdown 2012[6]

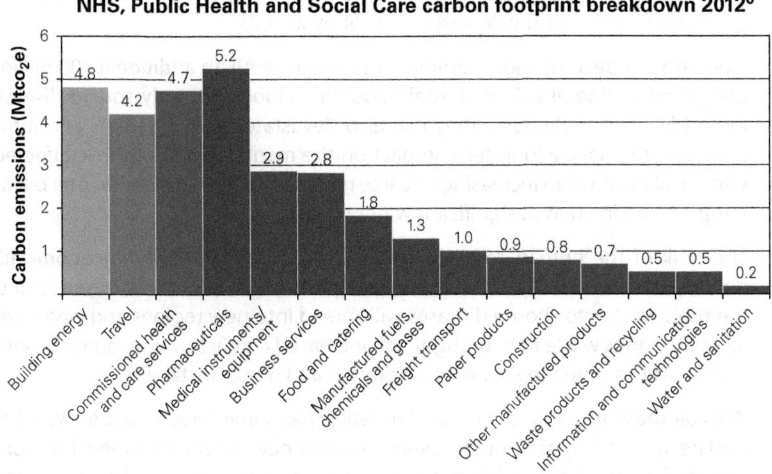

All of the above are major areas of financial cost to healthcare as well as being carbon intensive, demonstrating the close relationship that can exist between saving the planet and saving money.

The scale of healthcare's carbon footprint is something of which few leaders or clinicians are aware. When given the facts, the instinctive reaction of many is often to say 'it's hard enough saving lives, now you want us to save the world as well?' Well, yes. Because paradoxically healthcare will be among the primary victims of this problem as well as a leading perpetrator.

The Link Between Emissions and Illness

First, polluted air kills. Respiratory diseases such as COPD are the third most common cause of death globally and are exacerbated by poor air quality.[7] So too is asthma, an increasingly common conditions that is often lifelong and expensive to treat (ironically, inhalers are among the single most carbon-intensive healthcare product, making up around 8 per cent of the NHS's total greenhouse gas emissions[8]). Anyone who has visited one of China's major cities when the smog is present will understand the threat that air pollution poses to health. Outdoor air pollution has been estimated to contribute 1.2 million premature deaths every year in China, the fourth leading risk factor for loss of life expectancy (with indoor air pollution the fifth).[9]

Second, higher temperatures also kill. The 2003 European heatwave led to around 70,000 excess deaths across the continent.[10] Such events will become more common, for example Australia (which already has the world's highest rate of skin cancer) is predicted to see an increase of 'dangerously hot' days from an average of five per year now to 45 per year by 2070.[11]

Flooding will become more common and severe, with an additional 100 million people becoming at risk of coastal flooding.[12] Floods not only spread disease, loss of life and livelihoods, they can also devastate health systems and infrastructure and have a long-term impact on the mental health of those affected. Water will become an increasingly scarce resource, with an estimated one billion people living in areas of significant water stress by 2030.[13]

The bulk of the human cost of climate change will fall on less economically developed countries that are less able to cope and who have contributed least to the problem. Vector-borne diseases will spread into new regions and water and food shortages will lead to drought and increased conflict over resources. These, in turn, will combine to spur mass migration and global instability.

With all these impacts it is understandable that some have called for WHO to declare a fourth global public health emergency (following swine flu, polio and Ebola) until the world finds a more convincing response to the scale of the threat.[14] WHO has shown some leadership on the issue but the impact has been limited. Of all industries, healthcare should be in the vanguard of the low-carbon revolution; instead it has been among the most resistant to change.

The net impact of healthcare on society is overwhelmingly positive. However, we must recognise that there are costs as well as benefits. The concept of 'value-based healthcare' – where health outcomes are weighed against the cost of securing them – has spread around the world in recent years. In reality, though, healthcare leaders tend to calculate cost only from an economic perspective, ignoring social and environmental externalities such as landfill, wasted water, loss of biodiversity and greenhouse gas emissions. There is a price to lives in the future of saving lives now.

What is the true value of each healthcare intervention being provided today? We currently have no idea, partly because it is complex but primarily because it is not in the interests of very many organisations to know the answer. Other industries have shown that it is feasible to find out. Puma, the sportswear company, for example, now audits its business based on a triple bottom line that assesses the economic, social and environmental impact of its products across the whole supply chain. KPMG has a methodology called 'True Value' which similarly calculates costs and benefits across these three domains.[15] This can give a new perspective on the value of a project, substantially increasing or decreasing the projected benefits of a scheme based on its true value to a community's economic, social and environmental wealth.

Highly regulated markets such as mining and energy are beginning to think about their businesses more and more this way, as environmental costs are increasingly being converted to economic ones through tighter legislation. It would be fascinating to apply these kinds of holistic valuation methods to a decision about hospital reconfiguration or health service redesign, but it would be a brave leader indeed that justified a service change on the basis of environmental benefits, no matter how rational that is in reality.

Sustainable Health, Sustainable Planet

Fortunately, in all sorts of areas the economically sustainable model for healthcare is also the environmentally sustainable one. As the King's Fund has observed, to a large extent the changes needed to improve environmental sustainability are the same as those needed to deliver quality improvements and financial sustainability.[16] This triple bottom line pulls together in the direction of reducing waste, shifting care towards prevention and early intervention, and ensuring that treatment is right first time.

The NHS Sustainable Development Unit has identified 29 'best buy' solutions that, if implemented across the NHS, would simultaneously save £180 million and over 800,000 tonnes of CO2 per year.[17] These include smarter drug management systems to reduce waste, cutting down on medical packaging, installing combined heat and power generators in hospitals, and fitting better insulation into buildings.

Efficiency measures like these have enabled the Mayo Clinic in the US to reduce its energy consumption by 36 per cent since 2006,[18] a huge achievement in terms of cost and carbon when you consider that US hospitals currently spend a collective US$8.5 billion on energy per year.[19] Larger-scale schemes are active across the US, such as the Practice Greenhealth network of which 1,000 hospitals are members, as well as countries such as Thailand whose 'Green and Clean' programme is improving standards of energy use, waste production and food procurement across the health providers.

Some suppliers are also trying to play their part. Novo Nordisk is attempting to green the production of pharmaceuticals that make up such a large proportion of health-care's carbon footprint. It has consistently lowered its energy usage well beyond European efficiency targets by investing in hydroelectric and wind-powered factories as well as making them more efficient. It has also created enzyme technology that allows chemical reactions needed for production to take place at lower temperatures.

These win – wins are helpful, but even if they were adopted across the world's health systems they wouldn't come close to achieving the scale of change needed. To limit global temperature rises to a relatively 'safe' level the EU has agreed that its emissions need to be cut by 80–95 per cent by 2050, compared with 1990 levels.[20] Yet, this is at the same time as health systems in emerging economies realise their burgeoning ambitions for development and growth. If they follow the same models of care as the West, any savings by high-income countries will quickly become futile.[21]

Health and Social Care England Carbon Footprint[22]
CO_2e baseline from 1990 to 2025 with Climate Change targets

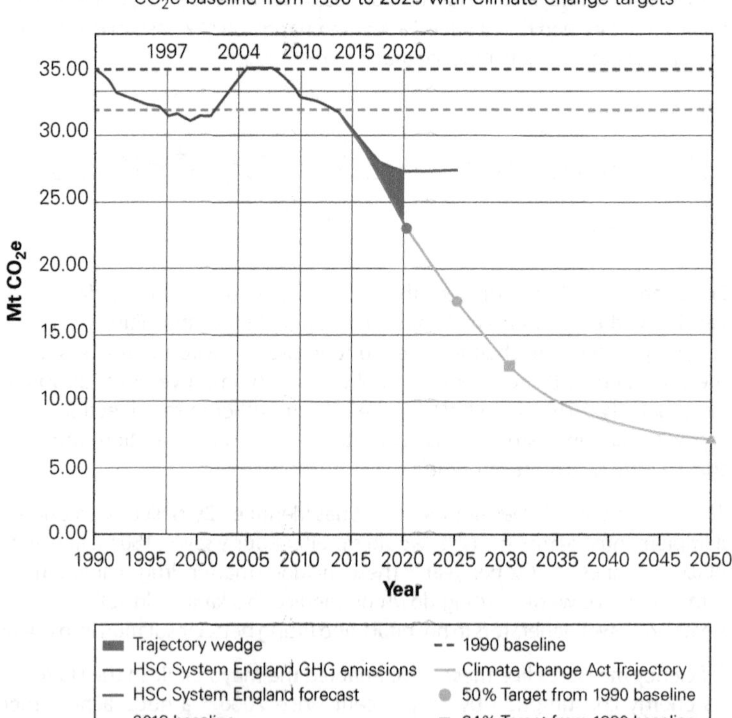

So, to achieve the level of transformation needed, health systems must focus not just on efficiency – doing things better – but a much more fundamental revolution in care – doing better things. Fortunately, when we look at what kinds of system would be able to deliver better population health at a fraction of the carbon cost, they look remarkably similar to the systems that many leaders have recognised as the solution to long-term sustainability in terms of quality and cost.

This starts with a much greater focus on prevention and health promotion, as the best way to make an activity more efficient is to not need it in the first place. In all kinds of ways, the high-carbon lifestyles that damage our planet are also damaging our health. Our diets, for example, are an increasing cause of heart disease, diabetes and certain cancers. We transport our food long distances so that supply chains are opaque and undermine strong local communities and economies.

Physical inactivity causes around 3.2 million deaths per year[23] and is a major economic cost to society, particularly in the rising trend of obesity that already is estimated to cost US$2 trillion annually.[24] Living environments and working patterns that discourage physical activity mean most people in developed economies live sedentary lifestyles. A 10 per cent increase in physical activity in the UK would save 6,000 lives and £500 million per year,[25] yet countries continue to invest disproportionately in infrastructure that promotes motorised transport rather than walking and cycling.

I can think of few payers or providers that have been bold enough to invest in green spaces for their communities, yet we know this has a major impact both on activity and the productivity of the workforce. KPMG research in the Netherlands showed that through reduced health service use, lower absenteeism and improved mental health, the scaling up of green spaces programmes to 10 million people would produce net financial benefits of €400 million.[26] Green spaces capture carbon through plants and the soil.

Prevention also involves keeping people with diseases healthy, so that they don't need more costly and invasive interventions. Those thinking about healthcare from financial, quality and environmental sustainability perspectives all see telehealth and telecare as critical enablers to better systems. If patients with chronic conditions can be monitored in real time from home, for example, we not only reduce the need for travel to and from consultations but can also intervene earlier and know with far greater certainty when care is required and when it isn't.

Technology can also help with the focus on empowering patients and carers to manage their own health better. We know that properly informed and involved patients will often choose less invasive and expensive treatments, resulting in the same or better outcomes at less cost. Shared decision-making protocols for elective surgical procedures, for example, have been shown to reduce demand by an average of 21 per cent while producing a better patient experience and no adverse impact on health outcomes.[27]

Looking at low- and middle-income countries, perhaps the biggest single win-win for healthcare and the planet is to improve access to maternal, child and family health services. Population growth has been a major factor in the growing emissions of the twentieth century, yet as nations develop and child mortality improves, without exception countries' birth rates drop. Safe birth and family planning services will help to control the world's population growth to a more sustainable level.

Conclusion

So, to any who remain sceptical about the reality of climate change, I propose this vision. Imagine for a moment that global warming has all been a hoax – the greatest scientific miscalculation since the flat-earth theory. We would still have created a more active, resilient, cost-efficient, self-sufficient, empowered, convenient and health-promoting society. As mistakes go, I'll be more than happy to hold my hands up.

References

1 Costello et al., 'Managing the health effects of climate change,' *The Lancet*, 373 (9676), pp. 1693–733 (2009).

2 KPMG International, Care in a changing world (KPMG, 2012).

3 KPMG (2012).

4 NHS Confederation, Taking the temperature: Towards an NHS response to global warming (NHS Confederation, 2007).

5 NHS Sustainable Development Unit for the NHS, Public Health and Social Care, Carbon footprint update for the NHS in England (NHS SDU, 2013).

6 Sustainable Development Unit for the NHS, Public Health and Social Care, NHS, public health and social care carbon footprint 2012 (SDU, 2014) p.6

7 World Health Organization statistics, 20 leading causes of death 2000–12 (WHO, 2014).

8 Hillman et al., 'Inhaled drugs and global warming: Time to shift to dry powder inhalers,' *BMJ*, 346, f3359 (2013).

9 Global Burden of Disease data (*Lancet*, 2010).

10 Robine J.M. et al., 'Death toll exceeded 70,000 in Europe during the summer of 2003,' *Comptes Rendues Biologie*, 331, pp. 171–8 (2008).

11 Global Climate and Health Alliance, Climate change: Health impacts and opportunities (GCHA, 2014).

12 GCHA (2014).

13 KPMG International, Future State 2030 (KPMG, 2014).

14 Godlee F., 'Climate change: WHO should now declare a public health emergency,' *BMJ*, 349, g5945 (2014).

15 KPMG International, A new vision for value (KPMG, 2014).

16 Naylor C. and Appleby J., Sustainable health and social care: Connecting environmental and financial performance (King's Fund, 2012).

[17] NHS Sustainable Development Unit, Saving carbon improving health: Update NHS carbon reduction strategy (NHS SDU, 2010).

[18] Mayo Clinic, Going Green, from http://mayoclinichealthsystem.org/locations/eau-claire/about-us/going-green.

[19] KPMG International, Care in a changing world (KPMG, 2012).

[20] European Union, Roadmap for moving to a low carbon economy by 2050 (EU, 2011).

[21] NHS Sustainable Development Unit for the NHS, Public Health and Social Care, Carbon footprint update for the NHS in England (NHS SDU, 2013).

[22] Sustainable Development Unit for the NHS, Public Health and Social Care, Sustainable, resilient, healthy people and places: A sustainable development strategy for the NHS, public health and social care system, (SDU, 2014) p.19.

[23] Hosking et al., Health co-benefits of climate change mitigation (World Health Organization, 2011).

[24] Dobbs et al., Overcoming obesity: An initial economic analysis (McKinsey Global Institute, 2014).

[25] NHS Confederation, Taking the temperature: Towards an NHS response to global warming (NHS Confederation, 2007).

[26] KPMG in the Netherlands, Green healthy and productive: The economics of ecosystems and biodiversity (KPMG, 2012).

[27] Stacy et al., Decision aids for people facing treatment or screening decision, Cochrane Database of Systematic Reviews: CD001431 (2014)

33 Ageing
Every cloud has a silver lining

It is a cause for celebration that we are living longer, but it is also the case that governments and societies across the world think they can put off the consequences. Ignoring problems and pressures usually makes them more difficult in the long run, so we should realise that ageing presents many positive possibilities – but only if we act sooner rather than later.

Since 1950, global life expectancy at birth has risen from 47 years to more than 67 and is expected to reach 75 around 2050.[1] In 2012 there were approximately 800 million people over the age of 60, making up 11 per cent of the world population. By 2030 they will number 1.4 billion (17 per cent of the global population) and by 2050 they will number 2 billion (22 per cent of the population).[2]

The current rate of ageing in low-income countries is much higher than in high-income ones. By 2050, 68 per cent of the world's population aged over 80 will be living in Asia, Latin America and the Caribbean.[3] China currently has around 220 million citizens aged over 60. This is forecast to soar to 500 million by around 2050, representing around a third of China's population,[4] and a fundamental shift in the global consumption of goods and services as a result.

This will create major shifts in global disease burden, none more so than dementia. There are currently around 44 million people living with dementia, with this figure rising rapidly and projected to hit 135 million by 2050.[5] Two-thirds of people with dementia live in low- and middle-income countries and the disease currently attracts barely a twelfth of the research funding dedicated to cancer, despite the fact that it already costs society perhaps twice as much.[6]

Globally the support ratio – the comparison between the number of people of working age (15–64) to those aged 65 or over – dropped from 11.75 working people for every older person in 1950 to 8.5 in 2012.[7] By 2050 it is estimated that there will be just 3.9 working-age people for every older person. The support ratio alone is a compelling reason for politicians to face up to the need for change as early as possible, as it portends a sharp decline in both informal family support and tax revenues to pay for care. There may never again be a more affordable time to prepare.

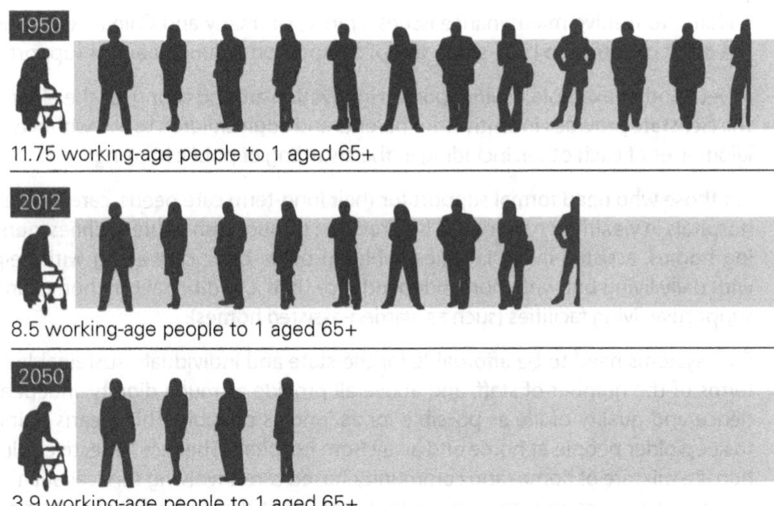

Number of people of working age (15–64) for each person aged 65+ globally[8]

Against all these pressures, however, I have seen many inspiring examples of people acting both quickly and innovatively to support older people to maintain health and independence. I illustrate six major trends below.

Boosting Informal Care

A growing number of governments are using both encouragement and compulsion to increase family support for elderly relatives.[9] One rather neat – but contentious – idea is that of Taiwan, which has changed inheritance rules so that children who have neglected their parents are prohibited from receiving inheritance. Hong Kong allows carers to pay a little less tax while its housing system supports multigenerational households.

India faces a big problem with children migrating to the cities and leaving their elderly with little support in rural areas. To tackle this, the Maintenance and Welfare of Parents and Senior Citizens Act 2007 requires children over 18 years to provide a minimum level of maintenance for their parents. If they fail to do so a struggling parent can apply to a local maintenance tribunal to obtain an order to provide a monthly allowance.

Singapore has gone even further down the route of forcing adults to care for their elderly parents. The Tribunal for the Maintenance of Parents ensures elderly parents can secure financial support while the Office of the Commissioner for the Maintenance of Parents provides a mediation service between parents and children to resolve maintenance issues. France, Germany and China are among the other countries to have some sort of compulsion around financial support.

In yet another example of Singaporean innovation around caring for the elderly, the city state provides incentives for parents and adult children to live within two kilometres of each other, including in the awarding of public housing.

For those who need formal support for their long-term care needs, care beyond hospitals in wealthier nations can be provided through sub-acute facilities, nursing homes, assisted-living facilities (which provide basic care along with help with daily living but with more independence than a traditional care home) and supportive living facilities (such as warden-assisted homes).

Care systems need to be affordable for the state and individuals, sustainable in terms of the number of staff, and above all provide as much dignity, independence and quality of life as possible for as long as possible. This means trying to keep older people at home and away from hospitals. The most effective solution is a mixture of home- and community-based care, involving services such as care management, nursing care, wound care, adult day-care and rehabilitation services, supported by informal caregivers. The proportion of elderly receiving care at home has been increasing in developed countries and currently stands at around 65 per cent across the OECD.

Communities as Carers

An innovation which offers great potential is the development of age-friendly communities. Retirement villages, often consisting of resident-owned homes built around facilities providing medical care, community services and entertainment, are an appealing but expensive approach. A more cost-effective alternative has been pioneered by Beacon Hill Village in Boston in the US.[10] This is a 'virtual village' where elderly residents and other volunteers in a neighbourhood, supported by a small core of paid staff, help one another with basic services such as transport, looking after the home and health and well-being.

In Japan, the Integrated Community-based Care System is aimed at ageing baby boomers. It provides services such as welfare, healthcare, long-term care and preventative measures within existing communities, accessible within 30 minutes. This community-based approach avoids the risk of creating isolated 'grey ghettos'.

The Role of Technology

The exploitation of technology in long-term care is still in its infancy, held back by the need for a stronger evidence base, the costs of installing technology across widely dispersed homes and the dependence on low-cost labour reducing the potential savings. But technology offers huge potential for increasing the efficiency of community care by allowing the real-time flow of data between care recipients and providers.

Remote monitoring systems help clinical staff to intervene only when necessary, while enabling them to respond to a developing problem before it becomes an emergency requiring hospitalisation. Health monitors worn externally or as implants are especially useful for people with cognitive and physical disabilities, such as by alerting care workers if a patient has suffered a fall.

Assistive technology will play an increasingly important role in the care of people with dementia. GPS systems can alert carers to someone leaving a building, while temperature, smoke and carbon monoxide detectors can be used to shut off gas or electricity supplies automatically or open windows. Medication dispensers can help people remember to take their medicines.

But technology has its downside; while for many it represents greater independence, for others it deprives them of valued human contact. The drive for efficiency must not lead to greater isolation.

Prevention and Self-Management

There is growing recognition of the value of prevention programmes aimed at older people, such as increasing physical activity, using medicines effectively, increasing health literacy and reducing the risk of falls. Prevention is now spreading into the areas of mental health and well-being, with increasing emphasis on, for example, preventing social isolation and training staff in public services, shops and transport systems to support the needs of older people, notably those with dementia.

But the best prevention and self-management approach is pursuing active and healthy ageing, by continuing to participate in the social, cultural and economic life of the community. But this is dependent on government help, such as by providing financial security, transport and other facilities which are old-age-friendly and support civic involvement.

The University of Southampton has attempted to quantify how well different countries achieve this goal by compiling an Active Ageing Index for European countries.[11] Nordic and Western European countries do best, with Sweden coming out top. Important factors include sustaining employment among older people and providing secure income for the retired.

Hospitals as Health Systems

Hospitals will, of course, continue to play a vital role in the care of the elderly. But they can only function in this new world if they are seen as one part of a system connecting acute care with specialist centres, nursing homes, primary care clinics, polyclinics, community centres, community hospitals, the patient's own home and nursing homes.

Doctors and other clinicians need to rethink how and where they perform their role to minimise the pressure on hospitals, maximise the effective use of alternative facilities which run at lower cost and exploit the potential of technology to keep patients well and managing themselves as much as possible. In the UK and the US this is variously referred to as the 'hospital at home' or 'the medical home' model. These approaches can reduce hospital admissions, improve care coordination, save money and improve the quality of life for the patient. In Singapore,

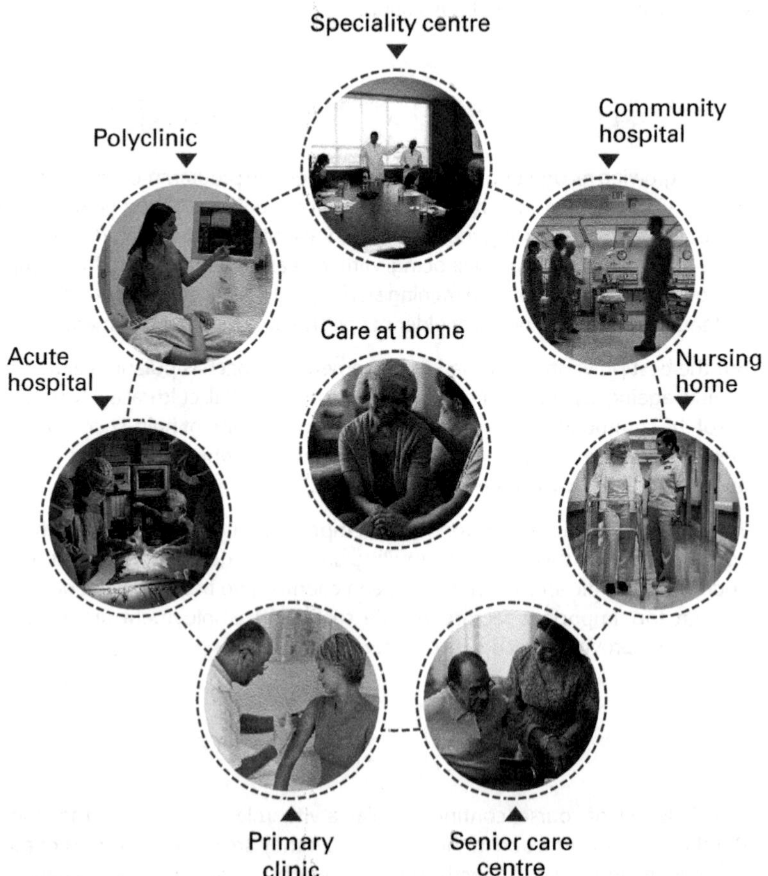

where the median age will be 55 by 2050,[12] the National Health Strategy is based around orchestrating the full continuum of care around the home. Rather than a 'closer to home' approach of shifting each level of care down to the next tier of providers, all providers are being asked to integrate their services into the home, so that even high acuity is now beginning to be delivered safely at home. This is requiring coordinated interventions with speciality centres, community hospitals, nursing homes, polyclinics and primary care.[13] It is an ambitious approach but, as KPMG's report *An Uncertain Age* describes, one rooted in a national conversation about ageing provoked by government and a real sense of urgency in the face of one of the fastest rates of ageing in the world.[14]

No Silver Bullet

Politicians, hospitals, care homes and home care providers will all have a major role to play. But even a cursory global survey of the actions governments and health systems are taking shows most are overawed. The scale of the challenge is simply too big and that is why so many are retreating into short-term fixes – baling out water rather than fixing the boat.

There is no one policy that will prepare a country for the pressures that come from rapid ageing. Transformation is needed in housing, food, finance, utilities, technology, transport, social support, exercise, entertainment and education sectors. No government is up to this task alone – the whole of society must be engaged to respond collectively.

I recently had the pleasure of addressing a meeting in the Netherlands in which KPMG convened a remarkable range of business leaders to discuss their contribution to 'healthy ageing'. Chief executives of a bank, a pension fund, a dairy producer, a construction company, a medical device maker, a pharmaceutical company, an academic medical centre and others were present. Our discussion revealed that there is a huge opportunity for the commercial sector to both lead and implement change around the world.

Merrill Lynch has estimated the 'silver economy' to be worth some US$15 trillion by 2020 (from US$8 trillion in 2010).[16] This growth is not just being fuelled by a larger number of older people – their behaviours are changing too. Whereas previous generations would have protected their wealth as their children's inheritance, there are signs that baby boomers are more inclined to use it to enjoy their (much longer) retirement. A recent survey from the UK showed that 30 per cent of over-55s planned to downsize in the 'near future', unlocking an average of £88,000 each. Forty-five per cent said they were planning to put this towards 'big ticket' purchases such as holidays and cars.[17]

So, the silver economy is attracting much interest for its commercial opportunities and our group of Dutch business leaders were full of ideas as to how they saw their contribution to ageing healthily. First, employers are improving their understanding about how to attract people into working longer – which keeps them healthier and more active, means there are more people in an economy earning and gets the most out of the valuable skills and experience that companies benefit from. This trend is already long underway, with the proportion of 55–64 year olds in work across the EU-27 increasing from 38 per cent in 2000 to 52 per cent in 2014.[18] Organisations such as Centrica in the UK have developed comprehensive strategies to retain older staff in employment and keep them engaged in their work. Even after retirement, organisations can continue to use older people's skills, as evidenced by Japan's 'Silver Human Resource Centres': a network of 800,000 members who offer part-time paid work such as translation, bookkeeping and maintenance work to businesses, public services and households.[19]

The commercial sector also has a major role to play in creating the housing and built environment to support independent living. The Netherlands itself has a leading example of a 'dementia village' which has attracted international interest.[20] Hogewey in Weesp is a community quite unlike any other. Residents – all of whom have severe dementia – live in groups of six in houses – each built to be reminiscent of eras which they will feel familiar with. There are those with décor and music from the 1950s and 1960s, and even one for aristocratic residents in which the carers behave like servants. They are actively involved in living as normal a life as possible – doing shopping and other activities as they are able.

Third, the technological opportunities of the ageing society – mentioned above – are attracting major investments from the medical device and wellness industries. Smart homes and wearables are already finding a growing market and if some of the brightest minds in Japan, South Korea and Singapore are to be believed, we will soon see a revolution in robotics for hospitals, homes and nursing facilities.

Fourth, service industries that have regular contact with older people can play a vital role in keeping them safe and well. In the 'dementia-friendly' town of Wels in Austria shop workers, postmen and public service staff have all been trained in the signs and symptoms of the disease and linked into services available if someone needs help.[21]

Finally, we may see a revitalising of the day-care sector in providing for societies searching for a middle ground between institutionalising people with care needs and having them live with their children. South Korea has seen an expansion of such facilities which offer formal services such as bathing and rehabilitation as well as social activities and meals.[22]

Conclusion

The challenge of caring for an ageing population is vastly greater than finding the money. It requires changes in attitudes, culture, social organisation, working patterns, housing and infrastructure, medical research, clinical training, and care organisation and delivery. While every country is talking about it and an exceptional few – such as Singapore, Japan and the Netherlands – are beginning to take concerted action, most of the world is doing far too little.

While the ageing population is almost invariably portrayed as a challenge, 'tsunami' or a problem, it is in reality an extraordinary opportunity. We have the chance to ensure millions of people live active, fulfilling and healthy lives that would have seemed inconceivable just a few generations ago while reshaping our healthcare systems around the needs of patients rather than the imperatives of healthcare institutions. But we need to act quickly.

Every year that is wasted while politicians and health leaders prevaricate is another tightening of the demographic screw. If we wait to make these changes until the drastic reductions in the ratio of working people to elderly become a reality, it will be too late. We have perhaps 20 years.

References

1 Hope P. et al., Creating sustainable health and care systems in ageing societies (Institute of Global Health Innovation, Imperial College London, 2012), p. 7.

2 Hope P. et al., (2012), p. 4.

3 United Nations, World population prospects: 2010 revision (UN, 2011).

4 KPMG International, An uncertain age: Reimagining long-term care in the 21st century (KPMG, 2013), p. 17.

5 Alzheimer's Disease International, Policy brief: The global impact of dementia 2013–50 (ADI, 2013).

6 Hope P. et al., (2012).

7 Hope P. et al., (2012).

8 Hope P. et al., (2012), p. 6.

9 Hope P. et al., (2012).

10 KPMG International, An uncertain age: Reimagining long-term care in the 21st century (KPMG, 2013).

11 United Nations Economic Commission for Europe & University of Southampton, Active ageing index 2014 (UN, 2015).

12 KMPG International, (2013), p. 9.

13 KPMG International, Staying power: Stories of success in global healthcare (KPMG, 2014), p. 17.

14 KPMG International, (2013), p. 38.

15 Ministry of Health of Singapore, Unpublished.

16 Nahal S. and Ma B., The silver dollar: Longevity revolution (Bank of America Merrill Lynch, 2014).

17 Prudential, Downsizing index (Prudential, 2014).

18 European Union statistics, Employment rate of older workers, aged 55–64 (EU, 2014).

19 International Longevity Centre, Japan's silver human resource centres (ILC, 2014).

20 Henley J., The village where people have dementia – and fun (*The Guardian*, 27 August 2012).

21 Rodrigues R. et al., Active and healthy ageing for better long-term care: A fresh look at innovative practice examples (European Union and Ministry of Health of Czech Republic, 2013).

22 Rodrigues R. et al. (2013).

Conclusion

34 Conclusion We wouldn't start from here

The dramatic increase in life expectancy during the twentieth century ranks as one of our greatest achievements. Sanitation, clean water, education, vaccinations and medicine have all played a part but the growing role of healthcare systems in helping the human race enjoy greater longevity should not be underestimated. Human beings have lived for approximately 8,000 generations but it is only in the past four or five that life expectancy has increased significantly. In the Bronze Age, average life expectancy was less than 30 years and it now stands at just over 70 (from Japan at nearly 84 years down to Sierra Leone at 38). Healthcare has made a significant contribution to the development of humankind, so why change a winning formula?

It is precisely because of longevity that our health system needs to change again. As people age, more chronic diseases affect our bodies, and our lifestyles – at least in the West – encourage this. If the twentieth century marked the high point of healthcare, the twenty-first century should herald the age of health. That's not to diminish the role of hospitals and healthcare systems but they will have to change if individual and population health are to be paramount. So, we should celebrate what we have achieved while preparing ourselves for the next big transformation: to healthy living.

We wouldn't start from where we are, knowing what we now know. It is difficult to transform institutions, professions and infrastructure that have developed over centuries and absorbed huge amounts of time, money and power. Health system and political leadership has never been more important. In this concluding chapter, I want to look at what we can change today while looking out for near-future trends that show great promise for tomorrow.

Universal Healthcare

We need to acknowledge that even today large parts of the world's population do not have access to universal healthcare. At best, only 40 per cent of the 192 countries in the world have it in some form.[1] As global wealth grows and becomes more polarised it is even more important for our political leaders to think long term and global and not always short term and national. It has been estimated that by 2016 half of global wealth was in the hands of the world's top 1 per cent.[2] This polarisation is not good for health: rich and poor alike. For example, a vaccine for Ebola could have been found years ago but it was considered by rich countries to be a disease of the poor, and the African poor at that. It is only because of our globalised and ever more connected world that richer countries became alarmed as infected people crossed their borders and large-scale trials seemed to begin almost overnight.

As BBC Economics Editor Robert Peston said: 'What the preventable tragedy of Ebola shows is that in a globalised world the interests of rich and poor are frequently the same – although it is hard for businesses to recognise this mutuality of interest when driven to make short-term profits.'[3] We have seen that political will, managerial skill, time and money are needed to secure universal healthcare, but it is a wise investment in our collective future.

Which Funding System is Best?

Let's assume the case for universal healthcare has strong moral, economic and political persuasion. The real obstacle, besides political will, is money. Across the world, a strong political and ideological debate is taking place about how best to finance universal care and fund health services. As we have seen, it is a difficult issue on which to pass judgement as all health systems are a product of their society, its norms and culture. Different systems are funded through different means: general taxation, social insurance, employer contribution, employee levy or international aid, grants, charitable donations and sin taxes. Globally, according to the OECD, the average ratio between public and government sources and private contributions stands at 72 per cent and 28 per cent respectively.

The debate about universal healthcare is frequently confused with the ability to pay. Universal (available to all), comprehensive (access to a full range of medical services) and free at the point of delivery (the ability to reclaim full costs or not pay directly for care received) have very different meanings depending on which country you live in. Germany first started the quest for universal care in the late nineteenth century through social insurance while Britain developed the first modern universal health system after the Second World War through a combination of progressive taxation and national insurance.

More recently, the rapid development of universal healthcare in Asia has seen a blend of employer–employee schemes, government subsidies and patient co-payments. I have been impressed with the tenacity, drive and purpose of the universal health systems created in Japan, Singapore, Korea and Hong Kong. They have high life expectancy (from 80 to 84 years) for modest costs (between 4 per cent and 9 per cent of GDP). South Korea achieved universal healthcare in

12 years, a remarkable feat of social policy and political will. However, in all these Asian cases, patient co-payments are high and would not necessarily be tolerated in parts of the West. Indeed, even in the Asian countries mentioned, there is growing public alarm at the direct costs of healthcare.

This is the fundamental point. There is no such thing as free healthcare; it is only a matter of who pays for it. Politics is the imperfect art of deciding 'who gets what, how and when'. High personal contributions create financial hardship for families, suppress spending power and slow economic growth while high government spending pushes up taxes, burdens business and acts as a brake on economic growth. There is merit and weakness in both these arguments but, to my mind, there is a long-term trend that charts a way through these ideological positions.

While there are good insurance-based health systems, for example in Switzerland, Germany, France and the Netherlands, they all spend higher amounts on healthcare at 11 per cent to 12 per cent of GDP. But a single or dominant pricing system and dominant payer seems to keep quality and access high and costs down for the population at large. This is a good trend for healthcare because it may enable additional funds to go into other areas such as education and economic stimulation that also contribute to health and well-being. We have already seen that there is little consistent correlation between high health spending and high health status but we do know that many non-healthcare factors contribute to well-being and improved life satisfaction.

Countries with a single-pricing system or dominant payer seem to have good life expectancy, modest costs, good access and lower patient co-payments. Sweden, Italy, Norway, Denmark, the UK, Japan, Spain and New Zealand all have life expectancy at around 80 plus years for around 9 per cent of GDP or lower. Insurance systems provide a little more choice and convenience but the benefits across the population at large do not outweigh the extra costs incurred. I have seen how insurance systems all too quickly pass medical cost or price inflation on to customers and consumers. While advances in care are sometimes more speedily implemented, costs are passed on more quickly. The direct, imperfect and asymmetrical relationship between the insurer and individual usually means the patient loses out.

In a single or dominant payer and pricing system, innovation can be slower but downward pressure is put on providers and suppliers which helps the population at large over time. In the long run, a dominant payer and pricing system is more able to pursue the triple aim of better health, better care and better value for the population at large.

The Perils of Fee-For-Service

If a dominant payer or pricing system keeps costs down, nothing less than a fundamental transformation of the payment system needs to occur if value is to increase. Crudely speaking, value is the patient outcome of healthcare divided by the costs. Most of the developed world and a worryingly high proportion of the developing world have a system which pays a fee for service.

This originated in the way that apothecaries and doctors received payments for services provided and was somewhat institutionalised in the move towards driving payments by disease diagnosis (diagnosis-related group system) in the last two decades of the twentieth century. While that system is good at driving volumes of care provided by independent practitioners or organisations it is not an ideal method for creating value. Instead, Porter and others have argued that integrated practice units, which look at diseases across clinical pathways and settings, are more responsive to patient and population needs. In KPMG's research on value-based care and accountable care organisations, even straightforward procedures such as hernia repair, hip replacement and hysterectomy require the collaboration of clinicians in different care settings such as rehabilitation, pain management and structured exercise.[4] Fee-for-service hampers such integration and is poor at controlling costs.

Integrated Care

With chronic conditions and an older population, multi-morbidity aged care accounts for more than half of the typical caseload of hospitals KPMG works with in high-income countries and more than 70 per cent of occupied bed days. Studies from across multiple developed systems typically show that between 20 per cent and 25 per cent of all patients could be cared for in different settings, quite frequently at home. What would happen to the airline industry if a quarter of passengers were routinely sitting in the wrong aeroplane?

Currently, in most instances, improving chronic care reduces admissions through active disease management in the primary care setting. But this often leads to a virtual stalemate since hospitals have no incentive to lose patients and income, and primary care providers have little incentive to undertake this extra work without extra resources or compensation. As Paul Batalden has said: 'Every system is perfectly designed to achieve exactly the results it gets. Sadly, all too often that means suboptimal quality, waste and frustrated professionals and patients.'[5]

It is not beyond the collective will and skill of healthcare professionals to design a better system. Ironically, I take some encouragement from the most costly and fragmented system in the world, the US. As the Affordable Care Act develops and access increases, there is an imperative to bend the cost curve. In New York State, for example, a five-year Delivery System Reform Incentive Payment (DSRIP) scheme seeks to align 25 self-organising Performing Provider Systems (PPSs) into integrated accountable care alliances that pursue value-based care. Across the world, I have found that if you want to give hospitals a way out of old business models you have to give them a way into a new care system. Hospitals should transform into health systems. In a recent KPMG survey, 93 per cent of healthcare leaders globally expected to see more bundled payment systems focused on value.

Transformations of this magnitude take will, skill and a lot of time and transitional funding. More importantly, they require a fundamental change in culture and a new form of health system leadership. I have already remarked that few individuals or organisations are rewarded and incentivised for sustainable, value-based population healthcare. The people running and working in hospitals care deeply about the 'triple aim' of better health, better care and better value but they are trapped in a system over which they feel they have little control. The good and the bad news is that their leaders feel the same.

I convened a global conference of 65 health leaders from 30 countries across six continents in 2014 and surveyed participants in advance. At the same time, KPMG crowdsourced across 50 countries to ascertain the feelings of ward managers, clinical directors and department heads. The results were illuminating. Across our global crowdsource community, 71 per cent believed that their own organisations required moderate or substantial change but 73 per cent believed their health system required fundamental change. Similarly, global healthcare leaders stated that 85 per cent of their efforts and focus were transactional (do things better) and only 15 per cent were transformative (do better things). Eighty-two per cent of global health leaders believed their health system would become more integrated in the next five years because fragmented care was hampering clinical effectiveness and operational efficiency. In its recent publication *Paths to Population Health*, KPMG outlines eight practical steps towards accountable and integrated care but the first precondition is a leadership style suited to partnership and a mindset that considers care system transformation as well as technical excellence in service delivery.[6]

Patient Power

Of course, transformation means nothing if patients are to remain passive beneficiaries of change. All industries that have transformed or have been fundamentally reshaped through competition, globalisation, technology and customer power have sought to harness the inherent value created by the consumer. And so it must be for health. Worryingly, in our global gathering of health leaders across 30 countries, 89 per cent believed that their own health systems were designed around their organisation's needs and not those of the patients they serve. Only 14 per cent of participants thought patients were becoming more active and activated. This lacuna is a fundamental issue for sustainable healthcare and a health-conscious society. Of course, responsibility must start and end with the individual but a well-aligned and incentivised health system can be a positive force. We know that activated patients consume between 8 per cent and 21 per cent less care, feel more satisfied and have better outcomes.[7] In work with payers, we have found that health coaching, care navigation and patient support groups produce tremendous rates of return, especially for high-volume chronic diseases. Inspired healthcare professionals such as Professor Bas Bloem in the Netherlands have demonstrated how patients can become activated through schemes such as Parkinson.Net, a patient-led, professionally supported network which has standardised care pathways and protocols that encourage participation and activation so that quality is improved, costs reduced and satisfaction sustained.

From God to Guide

Professor Bloem talks about the transformation of the medical specialist from 'God to guide'. It is a powerful concept and one which is still emerging. If patients are to become more activated and organisations more accountable, the wider healthcare workforce will need to change too. In KPMG's crowdsourcing work we surveyed hundreds of staff and while 88 per cent of care workers thought patient experience was a key performance indicator, less than half of health professionals had any objectives related to patient experience, let alone activation. Yet we know what patients want the world over. In our global research of patients groups, representing millions of patients across Brazil, Canada, the US, the Netherlands, the UK and Hong Kong, five key themes emerged in addition to care being delivered with dignity, courtesy and compassion:

Disconnect Between What Patients Want and What They Get: Five Dominant Themes:

1. 'See me and support me as a person, not as a condition or an intervention site'.
2. Patients want to be informed partners in care.
3. Fragmented care is harmful and wasteful care. Patients can feel abandoned – especially after discharge.
4. Patients want to be empowered partners in care.
5. In some countries, securing responsive access to care is a fundamental priority.

Staff in Control

While unleashing the potential for patients to become active partners in care is enormous, I believe that the increased motivation and improved management of the health workforce is one of the most neglected areas in healthcare today. The trapped or unlocked potential of millions of people across health systems is enormous. As I travel the world, in nearly every conference I speak at, I ask the audience what percentage of their staff have meaningful objective setting and appraisals (with consequences, actions, development and training) which are aligned with their team's objectives. You may be shocked to learn that fewer than a third keep their hands up after just a fleeting discussion. How can people consistently and tirelessly deliver compassionate care if they are not cared for too? Ironically, the special status of caregivers is often used as an excuse to transcend normal management methods. Healthcare professionals need both more power and greater accountability for what they do.

If change is a human contact sport then we had best contact human beings. Organisational charts often juxtapose organisational health (so-called softer measures such as culture, staff well-being and organisational development) and organisational performance (the hard metrics of activity, margins, profit and loss or shareholder return). While you can perform better on one than the other for a limited time, in the long run the best organisations seek a blended balance. The same should run true for hospitals, health practices and health plans alike. Health organisations can become at least 15 per cent more efficient and effective through better appraisal, staff management and development. As we noted in Value Walks, there are five characteristics that separate the great from the good and the bad: a strategic focus on value for patients, empowered staff, process redesign, effective use of information, and management of staff performance.[8] Given that we have a looming workforce shortage, we need to broaden the skill base of our staff, encourage their flexibility to make work more attractive and reduce costly demarcations that do not serve patients' interests. In other industries this is seen as mission critical; the same discipline needs to be applied at industrial scale in healthcare.

In *Staying Power*, KPMG showed how global healthcare leaders believe that continuity is the secret to sustainable change.[9] The move to universal healthcare, value-based outcome payments, accountable care organisations, inspired system leaders, activated patients and a motivated workforce takes superhuman effort and, put together, represents nothing less than the transformation of the existing healthcare sector. There are, however, other disruptive forces at play which might also dramatically change the landscape in the next decade or so. These will not be applied equally or universally but they exist already and will become increasingly important. Let me provide just five examples.

Genomics and Personalised Medicine

Perhaps the most exciting development is in the area of the genome and precision or personalised medicine. It has been over 60 years since Watson and Crick described the structure of DNA, while the complete sequencing of the human genome was achieved in 2003. Sequencing the first human genome took almost 10 years and cost almost one billion dollars; now it can be done in a day for less than US$2,000 – and the cost continues to fall. All this is encouraging and there has been a fair amount of hype around the ability to use genomics for cancers, rare congenital diseases and infections. A healthy number of national agencies have been developed, such as the excellent Genomics England, to see how further scientific discoveries can be applied across the NHS for the benefit of all patients.

Indeed, there is a consensus that genomics will improve the efficacy of our treatments and ultimately find new causes and cures but the real debate centres on when and how. Jeffrey Bland, President of Personalised Lifestyle Medicine Institute, suggests that once we reach '$1,000 genome analysis' the cost of the test will be around the same price as more traditional diagnostic tests and procedures, so payers will find the business model more attractive.[10] He claims that the adoption of new genomic tests will transform medicine because 'we are moving from a medicine for the average to a medicine for the individual'. He adds: 'It doesn't take clairvoyance to see the future. The future will be the incorporation of personalized medicine into health care.' His enthusiasm is supported by those who believe in universal healthcare as they argue that no civilised country or health system could deny treatment once a person's genetic disposition is known, and stress that only very wide population risk pools could withstand the likely costs. Sadly, on my global travels, it is the highly affluent with specialised health plans who seem to be taking advantage of personalised medicine at present.

I believe that genomics and personalised medicine does have a bright future this century because it will further challenge a health system which is currently centred on illness and not predictive and preventive well-being and lifestyle management. The way for healthcare payers to prove its worth will be to concentrate on high-risk groups in the first instance and design new healthcare delivery services around them to demonstrate much better value and an acceptable return on investment.

Mobile Health

Other industries will also disrupt healthcare. There are more than five billion mobile phones on the planet and they are already playing a transformational role in extending access to health. In India, KPMG has worked with a number of communication and information technology companies to create an integrated and personal care service for less affluent patients. The entire value chain is extremely lean. It starts with a small number of doctors (usually general practitioners) and nurse practitioners working in call centres supported by established clinical algorithms. Patients can access the service via their mobile phone network and pay the care service operator a small fee per call or monthly subscription. They call the centre and where possible a diagnosis is offered. Patients can then access their local pharmacies to obtain drugs or other services in low-cost settings. Many telecommunications companies are looking to expand way beyond their traditional customer base and see healthcare as a massive opportunity. There are a number of examples of telecoms companies buying doctor-run call centres which use high-contact, high-tech techniques to maintain close relationships with their customer and patient base. For example, Australian telecoms giant Telstra has invested over AUS$150 million in acquiring mobile health firms. It recently announced that it would launch a direct-to-GP telehealth service called ReadyCare, partnering with Swiss GP firm Medgate. As Eric Topol has said: 'Nearly anything we can do in medicine can be done remotely.'[11]

We have seen that mobile phones have been particularly beneficial where infrastructure is limited in Africa. As mobile devices become increasingly common throughout the continent, their potential in delivering better healthcare is being exploited by pharmaceutical firms such as Novartis. For example, patients would previously travel to far-off health clinics only to find that the medicines they needed were no longer in stock. Today, around 27,000 government health workers in Uganda use a mobile health system called mTRAC to report on medicine stocks across the country. Novartis is also working on an m-health pilot in Nairobi and Mombasa in Kenya to understand the supply chain cycle and ensure medicines reach patients in need. Pharmacists register their patients for surveys via SMS. The results help map out where patients are located in order to redistribute medicines to areas where they are most needed.

Apothecaries

If the telecoms industry is moving into healthcare then supermarkets and retail pharmacies are also mobilising. Although this is a relatively recent phenomenon, its roots can be traced back to 2600 BC and ancient Babylon where the first apothecaries were identified. Their name was derived from *apotheca*, meaning a place where wine, spices and herbs are stored (not unlike a supermarket today). By the mid-sixteenth century, apothecaries had become the equivalent of today's community pharmacists but their roles were more extended. Ironically, the mobilisation of supermarkets and retail pharmacies mirrors this old tradition to some extent but the scale and scope today is far greater.

In the US the giant supermarket chain Walmart intends to disrupt existing care pathways for minor ailments and other conditions while pharmacies and retailers such as CVS, Walgreens and Target want to expand aggressively in this area. With cheaper prices and quicker services, retail clinics are increasing exponentially and have doubled in number between 2012 and 2015.[12] For patients, convenience is a major attraction because they stay open longer than traditional doctor offices and surgeries, have shorter waiting times and cost less than hospital-run urgent care centres. They also have a relatively narrow focus on minor ailments and infections but accommodate large volumes of care. CVS runs the highly successful MinuteClinic to take the strain off other medical practitioners. The Association of American Medical Colleges estimates that physician shortages will soar by up to 90,000 by 2025, of which 31,000 will be primary care doctors.[13] Increasingly, retail clinics offer three types of care that have previously been fragmented: urgent, chronic and primary. Retail pharmacy is well placed to offer over-the-counter care while supporting patients to make the move from mobile health applications to self-care diagnostics (a growing market in its own right).

Similarly, research from the Royal Pharmaceutical Society in the UK has demonstrated that common ailments cost the NHS an extra £1.1 billion every year when patients are treated in accident and emergency or a GP surgery rather than a community pharmacy.[14] The research showed treatment results were as good as those from GPs and could reduce demand on stretched services by 18 million consultations per year – the equivalent of 5 per cent of the GP workload.

Wearable Technology

The latest wearable technology in the form of the Apple Watch can enhance fitness tracking and has other health-orientated capabilities (it can even tell the time). It has received near-universal acclaim but it was less than 70 years ago that this technology was introduced as a fantasy in a comic strip. Dick Tracy, the square-jawed, gadget-wearing detective, was created in 1931 and introduced the 2-Way Wrist Radio in 1946 to solve crimes. It was considered an extraordinary piece of fiction that captured the imagination of the public. It is now reality.

Today, the technology industry is creating a future of wearable devices that promises to entertain and captivate consumers, save them money and help them live healthier lives. Technology companies' interests in health and wellness have sparked the creation of myriad wearable devices, from fitness bands that monitor activity and sleep patterns to flexible patches that can detect body temperature, heart rate, hydration level and more. These devices produce data that can be used by consumers to manage their health and by healthcare organisations to improve care and potentially reduce costs through systems such as remote patient monitoring. Data generated by personal devices can be used by insurers and employers to better manage health, wellness and healthcare costs, and by pharmaceutical and life sciences companies to run robust clinical trials and capture data to support outcomes-based reimbursement.

It is estimated that half a billion people now use health applications[15] and consumers believe wearables can dramatically improve well-being, although some believe it is just a fad and experts have yet to find a sustainable healthcare business model. But the emergence of a personal consumer health market may allow these disruptive innovators into a different wellness space. Accenture estimates the consumer health market will be worth US$737 billion by 2018 and points to changing consumer behaviours, evolving healthcare policies and the digital revolution as the major forces driving growth.[16] Growing consumer awareness of health threats such as obesity will eventually drive a new demand for personal activation, support and monitoring. Accenture goes on to suggest that there will be industry convergence and says 'companies from life sciences, consumer goods, healthcare, telecommunications and high tech industries are all looking to capture the sizeable opportunity of this growing market'.

Some critics argue that wearable technology only really concerns 'the worried well'. These are relatively young people who are tech-savvy and health-conscious. While this may be true in part, the application of wearable technology can be applied to much broader groups in the future. In any event, consumer power is driving change.

Dignity in Death

> Being mortal is about the struggle to cope with the constraints of our biology, with the limits set by genes and cells and flesh and bone. Medical science has given us remarkable power to push against these limits… but again and again, I have seen the damage we in medicine do when we fail to acknowledge that such power is finite and always will be.[17]

In his moving book, *Being Mortal*, Atul Gawande reminds us of the limitations of medicine. My fifth and final innovation has much less to do with wellness and much more to do with well-being and dignity in death. Where possible, patients should be supported to die in their own beds. Sadly, patient power has yet to control and direct end-of-life care but this will change as the pressures of ageing increase and, in doing so, confront the culture and norms of society and medicine itself.

Longevity has brought many benefits to people and the population at large but most societies still don't talk about death and dying until it's too late. We know that people want a pain-free death, and more control, autonomy and independence in the final months and days of life. Death – like birth – is part of the full cycle of life but our over-medicalised model of care undermines dignity and compassion when it matters most. In England, fewer than 5 per cent of patients say they want to die in hospital, yet more than half end up doing so.[18] A National Audit Office study found that 40 per cent of deaths in hospital could have occurred at home or a hospice if sensible discussions and arrangements had been put in place beforehand.[19] Successive studies in the UK have demonstrated that hospitals are consistently rated by bereaved relatives as providing poorer care and lower levels of dignity and respect for people in the last days of life. End-of-life care outside hospitals is also estimated to be cheaper, with modelling work at King's College in London suggesting that costs could be reduced by £180 million each year across the NHS if awareness was greater and better services offered.[20]

The 2013 End of Life report for the World Innovation Summit for Health stated that 'how we care for the dying is a litmus test of a good health system and a responsible society'.[21] It went on to claim that only 8.5 per cent of all countries have integrated palliative care effectively into their wider health systems while 90 per cent of the world's morphine was used by just 16 per cent of the population thus 'revealing our historic emphasis on curative treatment while leaving the dying in pain'.

So, death, like life, requires the innovative mobilisation of patients, practitioners, families, communities, payers and providers to develop new models of care and attitudes to health in the twenty-first century. As Marie Curie, the first female scientist to be awarded a Nobel Prize said: 'Nothing in life is to be feared, it is only to be understood. Now is the time to understand more, so that we may fear less.'

References

1 McKee M. et al., 'Universal health coverage: A quest for all countries but under threat in some,' *Value in Health*, (16), pp. S39–45 (2013).

2 Oxfam, Wealth: Having it all and wanting more (Oxfam, 2015).

3 Peston R., Why extreme inequality hurts the rich (BBC News, 19 January 2015).

4 KPMG International, Contracting value: shifting paradigms (KPMG, 2012).

5 KPMG International (2012).

6 KPMG International, Paths to population health: Eight practical steps for achieving coordinated and accountable care (KPMG, 2015).

7 Hibbard J.H. et al., 'Patients with lower activation associated with higher costs: delivery systems should know their patients' "scores",' *Health Affairs*, 32, pp. 216–22 (2013).

8 KPMG International, Value walks: Successful habits for improving workforce motivation (KPMG, 2013).

9 KPMG International, Staying Power: Success stories in global healthcare (KPMG, 2014).

10 Bland J., Seeing over the health care horizon (*Huffington Post*, 23 December 2013).

11 Economist Intelligence Unit, Power to the patient: How mobile technology is transforming healthcare (EIU, 2015).

12 *The Economist*, Shock treatment (*The Economist*, 7 March 2015).

13 Association of American Medical College, Physician supply and demand through 2025: Key findings (AAMC, 2015).

[14] Royal Pharmaceutical Society, Pharmacists could save the NHS £1.1 billion by treating common ailments (RPS, 19 October 2014).

[15] KPMG in the US, Healthcare 3.0: Unlocking the value of big data (KPMG, 2015).

[16] Accenture, The changing future of consumer health (Accenture, 2014).

[17] Gawande A., *Being mortal: Medicine and what matters in the end* (Metropolitan Books: New York, 2014).

[18] Marie Curie, 1.4 million people could die in hospital against their wishes (Marie Curie, 27 April 2015).

[19] National Audit Office, End of life care review (NAO, 2008).

[20] Independent Palliative Care Funding Review, Funding the right care and support for everyone (Department of Health, 2011).

[21] Hughes Hallet T. et al., Dying healed: Transforming end of life care through innovation (World Innovation Summit for Health, 2013).

Key Statistics at a Glance

Country	Per capita health spending (US$)[1]	% GDP spent on health[2]	Change in % GDP spend on health (2003–13)[3]	Public spending on health as a % of total health spending[4]	GINI score[5]
Australia	6110	9.4	+0.7	66.6	0.33
Brazil	1085	9.7	+2.7	48.2	0.53
Canada	5718	10.9	+1.4	69.8	0.34
China	367	5.6	+0.8	55.8	0.42
Denmark	6270	10.6	+1.1	85.4	0.27
Finland	4449	9.4	+1.2	75.3	0.28
France	4864	11.7	+0.9	77.5	0.31
Germany	5006	11.3	+0.4	76.8	0.31
Hong Kong*	1716	6.1	0	48.7	0.37
Iceland	4126	9.1	−1.3	80.5	0.26
India	61	4	−0.4	32.2	0.34
Indonesia	107	3.1	+0.6	39	0.38
Israel	2599	7.2	−0.2	59.1	0.36
Italy	3155	9.1	−0.1	78	0.43
Japan	3966	10.3	+2.3	82.1	0.34
Malaysia	423	4	0	54.8	0.46
Mexico	664	6.2	+3.4	51.7	0.48
Netherlands	6145	12.9	+3.1	79.8	0.29
Norway	9715	9.6	−0.4	85.5	0.27
Portugal	2037	9.7	0	64.7	0.34
Qatar	2043	2.2	−1.9	83.8	0.41
Russia	957	6.5	+0.9	48.1	0.40
Singapore	2507	4.6	+0.7	39.8	0.43
South Africa	593	8.9	+0.3	48.4	0.65
South Korea	1880	7.2	+2.0	53.4	0.30
Sweden	5680	9.7	+0.4	81.5	0.27
Switzerland	9276	11.5	+0.6	66	0.29
UK	3598	9.1	+1.3	83.5	0.38
USA	9146	17.1	+2.0	47.1	0.44

*Some statistics for Hong Kong are taken from government sources and the Economist Intelligence Unit rather than those listed below, and may not be comparable

Sources

1 World Bank statistics, Health expenditure per capita (US$) (2013).
2 World Bank statistics, Health expenditure (% of GDP) (2013).
3 World Bank statistics, Health expenditure (% of GDP) (2003–13).
4 World Bank statistics, Health expenditure, public (% of total health expenditure) (2013).
5 OECD statistics, GINI coefficient of income distribution (2009–13).

Doctors per 1,000 people[6]	Life expectancy[7]	% obese[8]	% aged 65 and over[9]	Self-reported health (/100)[10]	Life satisfaction (/10)[11]	Country
3.3	82.2	28.6	15.0	85	7.3	Australia
1.9	73.9	20	8.0	69	7	Brazil
2.1	81.4	28	16.0	89	7.3	Canada
1.9	75.4	6.9	9.0			China
3.5	80.3	19.3	18.0	72	7.5	Denmark
2.9	80.8	20.6	20.0	65	7.4	Finland
3.2	82	23.9	18.0	67	6.5	France
3.9	81	20.1	21.0	65	7	Germany
1.8	83.7	21.1	14.0			Hong Kong*
3.5	83.1	22.8	13.0	77	7.5	Iceland
0.7	66.5	4.9	5.0			India
0.2	70.8	5.7	5.0			Indonesia
3.3	82.1	25.3	11.0	80	7.4	Israel
3.8	82.3	21	21.0	66	6	Italy
2.3	83.3	3.3	26.0	60	6.5	Japan
1.2	75	13.3	6.0			Malaysia
2.1	77.4	28.1	7.0	66	6.7	Mexico
2.9	81.1	19.8	18.0	76	7.3	Netherlands
4.3	81.4	23.1	16.0	76	7.4	Norway
4.1	80.3	20.1	19.0	46	5.1	Portugal
7.7	78.6	42.3	1.0			Qatar
4.3	71.1	24.1	13.0	37	6	Russia
2	82.3	6.2	11.0			Singapore
0.8	56.7	26.8	6.0			South Africa
2.1	81.5	5.8	13.0	72	7.5	South Korea
3.9	81.7	20.5	20.0	81	7.2	Sweden
4	82.7	19.4	18.0	81	7.5	Switzerland
2.8	81	28.1	19.0	74	6.8	UK
2.5	78.8	33.7	14.0	88	7.2	USA

[6] World Bank statistics, Physicians per 1,000 people (2010–13).

[7] World Bank statistics, Life expectancy at birth (2013).

[8] World Health Organization statistics, Body mass index >=30 (% of population) (2014).

[9] World Bank statistics, Population aged 65 and over (% of total) (2014).

[10] OECD Better Life Index, Average self-reported health (/100) (2014).

[11] OECD Better Life Index, Average life satisfaction score (/10) (2014).

Index

9781137496614

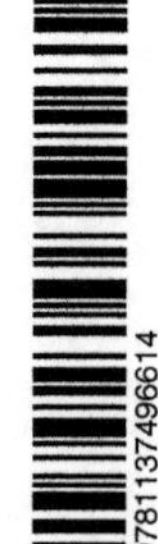